Rehabilitation Nursing

Foundations for Practice

D1395749

Edited by

Sally Davis MSc SRN SCM PGCEA DipMan
*Senior Lecturer: Rehabilitation, Rivermead Rehabilitation Centre,
School of Health Care, Oxford Brookes University, Oxford, UK and
Chair, RCN Rehabilitation Nurses' Forum*

Stephen O'Connor MA BSc PhD RGN RNT
Cert F. Ed.
*Lecturer in Nursing and Director of Adult Studies,
School of Nursing and Midwifery, University of Southampton, UK*

Foreword by

Catherine A. Tracey MS RN CRRN
*Director of Patient Care Management, Health Care Network, Manchester, NH, USA
Past President, Association of Rehabilitation Nurses*

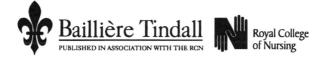

Baillière Tindall
PUBLISHED IN ASSOCIATION WITH THE RCN

Royal College
of Nursing

Edinburgh London New York Oxford Philadelphia St Louis Sydney Toronto

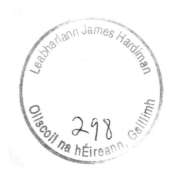

Baillière Tindall
An imprint of Elsevier Limited

First published 1999
  Reprinted 2001, 2003, 2004, 2005

ISBN 0 7020 2273 x

British Library Cataloguing in Publication Data
A catalogue record for this book is available from the British Library

Library of Congress Cataloguing in Publication Data
A catalogue record for this book is available from the Library of Congress

Note
Medical knowledge is constantly changing. As new information becomes available, changes in treatment, procedures, equipment and the use of drugs become necessary. The authors and the publishers have taken care to ensure that the information given in this text is accurate and up to date. However, readers are strongly advised to confirm that the information, especially with regard to drug usage, complies with the latest legislation and standards of practice.

The Publisher

 ELSEVIER your source for books, journals and multimedia in the health sciences

www.elsevierhealth.com

Working together to grow libraries in developing countries
www.elsevier.com | www.bookaid.org | www.sabre.org
ELSEVIER BOOK AID International Sabre Foundation

The publisher's policy is to use paper manufactured from sustainable forests

Printed in China
B/05

Contents

Contributors

June Bendall RGN ONC
Nurse Manager, Wolfson Medical
Rehabilitation Centre, London

Kathryn Bonney RGN ITEC
Senior Sister, Rakehead Rehabilitation Centre,
Nursing Development Unit, Burnley General
Hospital, Burnley

Iain Bowie MA BA(Hons) RGN DipN OND CertEd
Lecturer, Florence Nightingale Division of
Nursing and Midwifery, King's College, London

Lesley Crabtree BSc(Hons) RGN CertEdFE
Lecturer Practitioner, Department of Clinical
Geratology, The Radcliffe Infirmary and School
of Health Care, Oxford Brookes University,
Oxford

Sally Davis MSc SRN SCM PGCEA Dip Man
Senior Lecturer: Rehabilitation, Rivermead
Rehabilitation Centre, School of Health Care,
Oxford Brookes University, Oxford and
Chair, RCN Rehabilitation Nurses' Forum

Andy Elliott BA RGN
Freelance Nurse, Orsmskirk

Kaye Miller MSN CRRN
Rehabilitation Nurse Specialist, Devonshire
Hospital, London

Stephen O'Connor MA BSc PhD RGN RNT
CertFEd
Lecturer in Nursing and Director of Adult
Studies, School of Nursing and Midwifery,
University of Southampton

Mike Smith MSc RGN PG DipEd
Senior Lecturer, South Bank University, London

Gill Weaver RGN
Sister/Case Manager in Amputee Rehabilitation,
Rehabilitation Unit, Robert Barnes Rehabilitation
Centre, Cheshire

Susan A White BSc(Hons) RGN CRRN
Acute Elderly and Rehabilitation Nurse Specialist,
Barking Hospital, Essex

Hilary Whitelock RGN
Unit Manager, Alderbourne Rehabilitation Unit,
The Hillingdon Hospital, London

Foreword

The specialty practice of rehabilitation nursing is often misunderstood or underestimated. With the expansion of technology in healthcare, 'bells and whistles' often take our attention away from nursing that focuses on the whole person. Rehabilitation nursing is a philosophy of care: an approach to any individual who needs assistance with their ability to function in life. It is not a series of techniques or procedures alone. It is not practice that only occurs in a particular place or building. A rehabilitation nurse sees the potential of individuals whose illness or disability has altered their level of independence.

Also critical to the successful practice of rehabilitation nursing is the nurse's willingness to give up the authoritarian role that often inhabits many healthcare providers. Though this specialist nurse can offer his or her expertise, the true goal of any rehabilitation program is the transfer of knowledge, advocacy, and authority to the client.

Though rehabilitation nurses may work with individuals with varied clinical problems, there are a number of common threads that make this practice unique. Whether an individual is totally paralysed from a traumatic injury or is debilitated from an extensive acute illness, rehabilitation nurses focus first on function.

Maximising independence is the cornerstone of our practice. These efforts cannot occur without education. Everything from basic anatomy and physiology to the complex care of ventilator dependence must be explained in a way that each client can understand. These activities are based in the holistic practice of rehabilitation nursing. It is impossible to assist an individual to learn about their illness or disability and to maximise their independence without knowing them wholly. All human systems are inter-related and must be viewed in total. This is the complexity of rehabilitation nursing practice.

Anyone who has experienced a decline in function has most likely also experienced some sense of helplessness and loss of autonomy. Encouraging autonomy or empowering the individual to take control of their life is probably the most challenging but critical aspect of rehabilitation nursing. Regardless of the ultimate functional status of the individual, be they totally physically dependent or independent, the restoration of autonomy and empowerment is the true sign of rehabilitation.

Practising rehabilitation nursing is not for everyone. It is difficult physical and psychological work. In all of my years of practice, those who did it best had all of the following characteristics. In order to practise in a non-authoritarian role, the nurse must have self confidence. Being aware of one's own knowledge and skills, and continually seeking to advance them are traits common to excellent rehabilitation nurses.

In addition, I think it is near impossible to empower someone else if you are not empowered yourself. It also requires open mindedness to encourage individual expression and choices that reflect the client's values, not your own. This sometimes means the client rejects a nurse's education and advice. The rehabilitation nurse's role has a beginning and end. Though there may always be a nurse/client relationship, like parenting, there is a point when the rehabilitation nurse must let go.

Though all nursing requires compassion, the clinical situations that continually present themselves to rehabilitation nurses demand a high level of compassion. As soon as a nurse forgets the catastrophic nature of disability or illness, the necessary compassion is compromised. Rehabilitation nurses must rejuvenate and nurture themselves so they retain the generosity and compassion needed in this very special field.

The last but also very important characteristic the rehabilitation nurse must have is enthusiasm. Balanced with compassion, enthusiasm is necessary for small and big accomplishments. Though it was 20 years ago, I clearly remember my screams of joy when one of my patients, a 16-year-old girl with C 6 quadraplegia, catheterized herself the first time. We also had many tearful moments together but when the time was right, we cheered. Just thinking about this moment reminds me how special rehabilitation nursing is.

I had the pleasure of meeting many of the individuals involved in the publication of this book about two years ago. Their commitment to the specialty of rehabilitation nursing was evident then and now. The volunteer hours spent to educate and promote the specialty of rehabilitation nursing is inspiring. I was impressed with not only the nursing process chapters on rehabilitation nursing but also the space dedicated to the theory and models that serve as the foundation for our specialty. It isn't enough to know just the clinical techniques of rehabilitation nursing. Intelligent, thinking nurses need to practice within a theoretical framework. Likewise, that practice needs to be evidence based. Whether one is directly involved in research or not, all nurses need to constantly update their practice with research findings.

The contributors and editors of *Rehabilitation Nursing: Foundations for Practice* have written an excellent resource for all rehabilitation nurses. Your work is so critical to those we serve. Read it with enthusiasm and compassion.

Catherine A Tracey

Introduction

Rehabilitation nursing: a UK perspective

This book has been written in response to the need of nurses for an informed text on rehabilitation nursing. Awareness of rehabilitation generally has increased due to documents such as *The Health of the Nation* (DOH, 1992), and government directives to health authorities regarding reviews of their rehabilitation services.

This book is written at degree level and is aimed at pre-registration and post-registration nurses. It is general enough to be used in any health care setting, for example, acute clinical areas, the community, learning disabilities nursing and specialised rehabilitation centres.

The idea of this book was first identified by the Rehabilitation Nurses' Forum, which is affiliated to the Royal College of Nursing. The forum was originally formed in 1990 with the aim of providing an arena for rehabilitation nurses to share ideas and to raise the profile of rehabilitation. The forum has identified a 'philosophy' for rehabilitation nursing, on which the RCN publication *Standards of Care for Rehabilitation Nursing* (RCN 1994) is based. The philosophy identifies the following beliefs about rehabilitation and rehabilitation nurses:

- Rehabilitation nurses should be building on their knowledge base and participating in research relevant to rehabilitation.
- Rehabilitation should commence at the onset of illness.
- An interdisciplinary approach is essential if rehabilitation based on goal-planning is to achieve the best outcome for the client and family.
- Effectiveness and continuity in rehabilitation can only be achieved through the provision of a 24-hour/7-day-a-week interdisciplinary service.
- Clients are people with individual personalities and needs.
- Rehabilitation nurses have a role to play in educating nurses and other professionals in rehabilitation.
- Clients have a right to privacy, dignity and a right to say 'no'.
- Recreation, leisure and social interaction are important aspects of rehabilitation.
- Clients are entitled to have a high standard of care from a named registered nurse and named therapists.

- A framework is needed to assess, plan and evaluate care, which should be developed in partnership with the client and family.
- A health promotion focus is necessary to enable rehabilitation nurses to concentrate on health and wellness rather than disability and illness.
- Education should be ongoing and must cater for the specialist needs of rehabilitation for staff, clients and relatives.

In keeping with these beliefs, the main aim of this book is to provide an appropriate knowledge base for the development of rehabilitation nursing practice, addressing the main areas identified in the philosophy. It is hoped that the book will:

- stimulate and generate informed learning
- act as a springboard for further study and professional development
- act as a catalyst to promote change and stimulate innovation
- be used as a resource
- promote awareness of research related to rehabilitation
- enable nurses to be selective and critical in the application of research findings to practice
- provide nurses with a knowledge base to assess clients' rehabilitation needs, to plan and evaluate care
- enable nurses to identify rehabilitation principles as an integral element of nursing care
- be proactive in promoting rehabilitation as a multifaceted, complex, holistic, dynamic process.

The majority of chapters within the book have been written by members of the Rehabilitation Nurses' Forum, and all have been written with references to research and relevant literature, offering a critical and analytical view thereof. The relationship between theory and practice is recognised as being vital and is constantly demonstrated. Examples from practice in the form of vignettes illustrate this link.

The book is divided into three main sections: General Issues, Care Planning and Rehabilitation, and Issues in Rehabilitation Nursing. When discussing the whole topic of rehabilitation we realised that the potential for content was enormous. What to include and what to exclude? We felt that dividing it into three sections would assist in keeping a focus, and would also enable nurses to 'dip in and out' for areas of individual interest.

The aim of the first section of the book is to provide nurses with a background to rehabilitation and an understanding of theoretical frameworks and concepts. Section 2 is devoted to the nurse's role in rehabilitation, which is explored in the context of care planning and rehabilitation. Section 3 is concerned with specific issues in rehabilitation nursing and is intended to challenge thinking about rehabilitation issues which could be identified as controversial.

So, there is nothing left to say except enjoy the book, and we hope that it will provide you with the knowledge and enthusiasm to promote rehabilitation nursing in your area.

Sally Davis
Stephen O'Connor

References

Department of Health (1992) *The Health of the Nation*. London: HMSO.

Royal College of Nursing (1994) *Standards of Care for Rehabilitation Nursing*. London: Scutari.

SECTION

1

GENERAL ISSUES

1 Models and theories

Sally Davis, Stephen O'Connor

Key issues
- Definitions of rehabilitation
- Quality of life
- Activities of living
- Self-care
- Adaptation
- Other concepts and theoretical frameworks
- Views of disability

Introduction

The aim of this chapter is to challenge nurses' thinking about what rehabilitation is, and to provide them with a selection of frameworks which they can use to make sense of rehabilitation, and on which to base their own practice.

As a process, rehabilitation is complex, with a number of phenomena related to it, such as adaptation, stress, adjustment, independence, activities of living, self-care, motivation, illness, and wellness. It is not possible to explore all of these phenomena in detail in this chapter. Activities of living, self-care and adaptation are concepts which form the basis of the nursing models most commonly used by rehabilitation nurses, and it is these concepts which will be explored in more detail.

It is first necessary, however, to examine the term 'rehabilitation' and to explore the concept of quality of life, which can be identified as being the ultimate measure of rehabilitation.

Definitions of rehabilitation

Rehabilitation is not a new word, being used as far back as 1696 when it was described by the Oxford English Dictionary as 'an act whereby the Pope or the King by dispensation or letters restores those that are grown low in the world'. Throughout history, the word has been used in various contexts, for example, sending convicts to Australia in the 18th Century was part of a 'rehabilitation' process, and in 1941 it was reported that a military victory would be followed by the economic and democratic 'rehabilitation' of France and Germany.

The term rehabilitation can be applied to very diverse things, like crumbling buildings, convicted prisoners, frail old ladies or disgraced politicians, meaning to restore, to renovate, or to re-clothe an object of misfortune, so that it regains its previous function (Oxford

Medical Companion, 1994). From its Latin roots, habitation means to live, so rehabilitation would mean to relive, or live again.

In the literature, rehabilitation is defined in a number of ways. It is impossible to include them all here, so a variety have been chosen which reflect the general ambience of the majority of the definitions (see Box 1.1).

Box 1.1
Definitions of
rehabilitation

- An active process which seeks to reduce the effects of disease (in its broadest sense) on daily life.

    (Greenwood, et al., 1993)

- The whole process of enabling and facilitating the restoration of a disabled person to regain optimal functioning (physically, socially, and psychologically) as fully as they are able or motivated to do so.

    (Waters, 1986)

- A dynamic process in which a disabled person is aided in achieving optimum physical, emotional, psychological, social or vocational potential to maintain dignity and self respect in a life that is as independent and self-fulfilling as possible.

    (Lippincott, 1985)

- Re-activation – the encouragement of patients to be active witin their surroundings. Re-socialisation – the encouragement of physical and/or verbal contact by patients with peers, family and others. Re-integration – restoration of the patient to society and the regaining of status as a person.

    (Jackson, 1984)

- The restoration of an individual's ability to function as efficiently and normally as his condition will permit following injury, illness or accident. It involves re-education and retraining of those who have become partially or wholly incapacitated by such conditions as blindness, deafness, heart disease, amputation, paralysis.

    (Blackwell, 1994)

- Concerned with the intrinsic worth and dignity of the individual. It is therefore committed to the restoration of the disabled to a life that is purposeful and satisfying, one that allows each individual the opportunity to function adequately as a family member and as a member of society with the capabilities to meet the responsibilities of that society.

    (Licht, 1968)

- The process by which a person works toward a former level of functioning after experiencing some type of injury or the effects of a disease. Rehabilitation is achieved by relearning skills formerly mastered and by learning new ways to do activities one no longer can accomplish with previously learned skills.

    (Chipps, Clanin and Campbell, 1992)

- The combined and coordinated use of medical, social, educational and vocational measures for training or retraining the individual to the highest possible level of functional ability.

  (WHO, 1969)

- An educational, problem-solving process aimed at reducing disability and handicap.

  (Wade, 1990)

These definitions highlight certain defining attributes of rehabilitation, detailed in Box 1.2.

Box 1.2
Defining attributes of rehabilitation

Process	Rehabilitation is generally described as being a continuing process which is concerned with physical, social and psychological aspects. A process which should be active and dynamic, with the client taking an active part.
Restoration	Restore or restoration is used in terms of enabling the client to regain lost elements of their life, such as physical functioning or personal and social identity. It is also used in the sense of restoring the client to society or to a purposeful and satisfying life. To restore can imply that the emphasis of rehabilitation is on the client returning to their former life, rather than on adapting to their changed circumstances and learning new skills, which is the way it is meant in most of the definitions.
Effectiveness	Rehabilitation is described as promoting effectiveness or optimal functioning for the client.
Enabling and facilitating	Rather than a 'passive, doing for' process, rehabilitation is generally described as being an enabling and facilitating process, which is conducive to it being active rather than passive.
Learning and teaching	Rehabilitation is often described as being an educational process which enables clients and carers to learn new skills.

As well as being a process, rehabilitation can be identified as being a philosophy of care which should underpin all aspects of health care (Preston, 1994; RCN, 1994).

It is perhaps relevant here to mention the World Health Organisation's ICIDH (International Classification of Impairments, Disabilities, and Handicaps) (WHO, 1980) which suggests that conditions can be looked at on four levels. This framework is being used more and more in rehabilitation settings to address the totality of rehabilitation. Within this framework, the four levels identified are listed in Box 1.3.

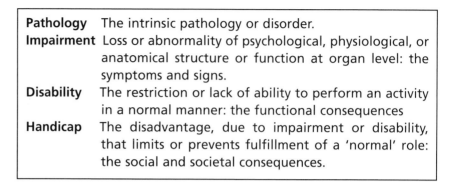

Pathology	The intrinsic pathology or disorder.
Impairment	Loss or abnormality of psychological, physiological, or anatomical structure or function at organ level: the symptoms and signs.
Disability	The restriction or lack of ability to perform an activity in a normal manner: the functional consequences
Handicap	The disadvantage, due to impairment or disability, that limits or prevents fulfillment of a 'normal' role: the social and societal consequences.

There are difficulties with the WHO model in identifying the differences between the levels. There is an implication within the WHO model that disability is the direct result of impairment, whereas rehabilitation therapists seek to minimise disability in the face of enduring impairment (Johnston, 1996).

It is important that rehabilitation is focused on the level of handicap rather than on disability. By focusing on handicap, rehabilitation will be concerned with the client's quality of life within society. If rehabilitation stops at the level of disability, then clients may have their level of disability reduced, but this will not necessarily mean that they can assume a quality of life which is acceptable to them. Rehabilitation is about much more than just the reduction of disability.

Quality of life

Quality of life can be considered as being central to any discussion of the individual experience of living with chronic illness or disability. Though an intuitive understanding of the concept is easily attainable, attempts to define the concept are more frequently than not either gross oversimplifications or clumsy tautologies. This section will not, therefore, debate the merits of various attempts to define the concept, but will briefly outline the breadth of the debate concerning a definition, and the inherent tensions within the practice as to the usage of the concept.

There is no doubt that the use of improved quality of life as a goal of rehabilitative care is reasonable. By definition, clients whose acquired impairments change their daily lives must live within an altered set of circumstances that affects what can reasonably be considered as their quality of life. That the individual should strive to gain an acceptable 'quality of life', though perhaps grossly altered, would therefore seem self-evident as a factor of their rehabilitation. The problems arise when attempts to operationalise the concept of quality of life are made. Attempts to move the usage of the concept (in terms of goal-setting and outcome measures) beyond the general to the specific causes problems not only of definition, but also in the daily practice of nurses.

Draper (1997) summarises in three main areas the problems that arise as a result of attempts to operationalise the concept. First, Draper states that the concept can be seen as either a subjective or an objective phenomenon. Secondly, the concept can be seen as either a feature of the individual or of populations. Thirdly, and perhaps most importantly for rehabilitation nursing, is the question of the possibility of the improvement of quality of life by outside interested parties. The rest of this section will concentrate on the first of Draper's questions regarding subjectivity and objectivity. For a fuller discussion of the others, the reader is recommended to explore Draper's full text (Draper, 1997) and also those of Brown (1997) and Baldwin et al. (1990).

To explore this debate, the approach taken by various authors to the breadth of the concept will be discussed. The subjective viewpoint is characterised by the views of Fraley (1992) who, while agreeing that the concept of quality of life is indefinable, points to the central feature being the different meanings that are expressed by individuals, due to their variable values and life situations. Fraley considers individual definitions to be based upon subjective criteria, such as 'past experiences, past successes, future goals and present self esteem' (Fraley, 1992). The nature of the criteria as defined by Fraley demonstrate the transient characteristic of the overall concept. Given such an approach to quality of life, the ability of the rehabilitation nurse to alter an individual's quality of life would appear to be limited to the realms of psychosocial counselling and general psychological support activities. Such activities have been identified by various authors as within the interventions of the rehabilitation nurse (Kirkevold, 1997, O'Connor, 1993, 1997; Waters, 1986, 1991).

In contrast to the above, the earlier approach taken by Diamond and Jones (1983) is of interest. These authors, while accepting that the concept of quality of life is closely related to the individual's personal values and judgements, argue that more objective criteria must also be considered. To this end, the authors discuss the applicability of characteristics such as functional status, in the guise of ability of the individual to self-care and participate in society, alongside socio-economic status, in the form of financial and material self sufficiency (Diamond and Jones, 1983).

The obvious difference between the two approaches is the addition in the latter of criteria that lend themselves to objective scaling, and therefore direct measurement. The addition of self-care activities as a major aspect of quality of life enables nurses and other members of the interdisciplinary team to believe that they can improve clients' quality of life by improving their self-care skills. Similarly, 'participation in society' can also be influenced by carers to the extent that the client's level of participation can be 'improved' in various ways. The possibility that such changes can then be measured and compared results in the logical extension of the approach such that aspects of, if not the totality of, quality of life can also be measured.

Therefore, by such seemingly small changes or additions to the breadth of criteria for a working definition of quality of life, the full range of objective scales and measures can be justified and therefore constructed. Such an approach when taken to its fullest extent produces the 'Quality Adjusted Life Year' or 'QUALY', a system of calculation which considers quality of life in terms of cost–benefit analysis. Such an approach to quality of life, although very influential in the 1980s, has now been severely criticised. For example, Cummins (1997) argues most effectively that such an approach is 'a bizarre notion that is based on invalid psychometric assumptions'. This may well be the case, but the point to be noted here is that over-emphasis on objective criteria inevitably dissociates the meaning of quality of life from the lived reality of the individual.

However, total rejection of all belief in the role of objective criteria would be an error. Given that a purist subjective approach to the concept of quality of life may well most accurately reflect the individual's comprehension of their experience, such an approach can also be seen to reject the impact of objective criteria, such as those anticipated by Diamond and Jones (1983). The application of objective criteria, such as the individual's ability in self-care activities and degree of social integration, does make intuitive sense, in the same way that the subjective approach does. The important point is not to allow the attractiveness of measures and scales to subsume the vital importance of the individual's subjective impressions.

Even though this section argues for a balance between the two approaches, the importance of objective measures of quality of life cannot be underestimated. These can be relatively simple measures such as the Barthel Index which, though not strictly defined as a quality of life measure, estimates various indices of self-care, and given Fraley's criteria can in some small fashion be accepted to estimate quality of life. The more complicated and specifically designed measures generally make use of broader sets of criteria, such as the five 'domain areas' put forward by Felce and Perry (1997):

- Physical well-being
- Material well-being
- Social well-being
- Emotional well-being
- Productive well-being.

These criteria can be considered as individual criteria, or as being constituents of quality of life, and therefore part of a single cumulative index. Such an index, even though complicated in construction, could be perceived as a gross oversimplification. However, the use of such indices is not uncommon, and can be seen to be of use when comparing definable groups against the population as a whole (Felce and Perry, 1997).

This section of the chapter has attempted to demonstrate the breadth of the concept of quality of life. The position taken by Felce and Perry (1997), that a definition that balances 'the five domain areas suggests that measurement of life conditions, subjective assessments about life and personal values are all relevant', would seem to be a reasonable one for the nurse involved in the very practical activity of rehabilitation.

Activities of living

The use of activity of living models has a well documented history in UK nursing, where it is recorded as one of the most popular types of model in clinical practice (McKenna, 1994; Mason and Chanley, 1990). Similarly, in a survey of stroke units (O'Connor, 1996), the most common models identified were activity of living models, such as those of Henderson (1966) and Roper, Logan and Tierney (1990), which were used in nineteen of the units. As the Roper, Logan and Tierney (RLT) is a linear development of the Henderson model (McKenna, 1997), it is the later model that will be discussed in this chapter.

Central to an understanding of the meaning and popularity of the RLT model is an appreciation of the nature of activities of living. Hoeman (1996) defines these as:

'all those things that people do in everyday life and with which people need help when they are unable to perform them independently'

The exact nature of these activities depends upon the individual's position on two independent continua: first, a continuum between total independence at one pole and total dependence at the other; secondly, a continuum between the new-born at one pole and the aged adult at the other. The independence/dependence continuum represents a dynamic process, along which individuals move in relation to their ability to control their own activities of living. Their exact position is affected by a number of factors that limit the individual's ability for maximum independence. Hoeman (1996) classifies these limiting factors as: first, the physical, psychological, and social environments; secondly, disability and disturbed physiology; thirdly, degenerative or pathological tissue changes; lastly, accidents.

The second continuum, that of life-span, is the most important factor determining individuals' abilities to undertake activities of living for themselves. This is essentially self-explanatory, in that individuals' ages will directly affect their ability to maintain their own activities, the most obvious example being the new-born, but all other age groups also have limiting factors. The sum result of these two continua is the nature of the person as perceived within the RLT model. The individual is considered as:

> *'an unfragmented whole who carries out or is assisted in carrying out those activities that contribute to the process of living'*
> (Roper et al., 1990)

The second most important concept is that of the nature of health within the model. Health is considered to be:

> *'the optimum level of independence in each level of activity of living which enables the individual to function at his or her maximum potential'*
> (Roper et al., 1990)

The important point in this definition is that health is considered to be a relative concept, not an absolute one. That is, an *optimum* level of independence is anticipated to allow function at an *optimum* level. This reflects a much more considered approach to the effects of the continua on the individuals' abilities and is an important feature of the model which will be returned to later in the chapter.

Closely associated with the above concept of health is the way the environment is perceived within the model. The environment is considered as:

> *'those circumstances that may impinge upon the individual as he or she travels along their life-span and cause movements towards maximum dependence or maximum independence'*
> (Roper et al., 1990)

The environment is seen as the engine of change, the mechanism through which the limiting factors defined above affect the individual. Such an approach should not be seen as a negative one, as the environment is also a liberating influence since it can also enhance independence.

The relationship of nursing to the above concepts lies in the situations that are implied in both the definition of the person and of health. In these definitions, it is anticipated that situations will arise, or are part of the life-span continuum, where the individual will not be able, for identifiable reasons to undertake the maintenance of all their own activities of living. Hence nursing is perceived as:

> *'a profession where the focus is to help the client to prevent, solve, alleviate or cope with problems associated with the activities of living he or she carries out in order to live'*
> (Roper et al., 1990)

The relationship between these key concepts of the RLT model can be seen in Figure 1.1. The figure highlights the principal theme

Figure 1.1
Diagrammatic representation of the relationship between the key concepts of the Roper, Logan and Tierney activities of living model of nursing

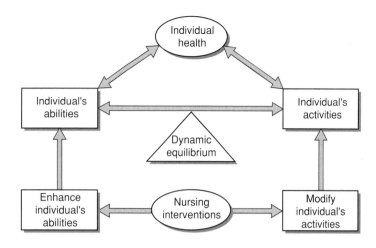

that underpins the model, that of balance or dynamic equilibrium between the individual's abilities and activities. The individual's health is a balance between their essential activities of living and their abilities to fulfil them. This balance is a dynamic equilibrium, since both the required activities of living and the individual's abilities are continually changing due to the effects of the environment: changes along the life-span and independence/dependence continua. The interventions of nurses are illustrated as attempting to help maintain or re-establish an equilibrium when such becomes unbalanced. This can be achieved in two ways, by modifying the activities that need to be undertaken, enhancing the individual's abilities to maintain their own activities or, in all likelihood, a combination of both. Such interventions would then re-establish an equilibrium that is once more under the control of the individual, and nursing intervention could be withdrawn.

Activities of living and rehabilitation

The fact that the RLT model is popular in rehabilitation could be seen to be a function of the fact that, as the model is popular in general nursing, it is transferred to the rehabilitation setting as a first option. This would seem to fit in with the results of the survey of stroke units (O'Conor, 1996) that demonstrated a particular pattern of models and changes of model. The most common models identified were activity of living models such as those of Henderson (1966) and Roper et al. (1990) which were used in nineteen of the units, and Orem (1991) in another eleven. The remaining four units used adaptation models, that of Roy (1990) in three cases, and an individualised model based on Roy in the final case. What was interesting to note was that there seemed to be a line of progression along which units developed, in terms of the model that they used. Many units added in their responses, that they were in the process of movement or development. In general, those using Henderson or RLT and contemplating a move were planning to use Orem and those using Orem and considering a shift were planning to move to Roy, although several planned to move from Henderson/RLT directly to Roy. The use of these models in practice would indicate that applicability is a matter of development by the nurses concerned. Only by the practical use of models can nurses develop a feeling for what is correct in their area of care. The movement from Henderson/RLT to Orem to Roy would indicate an increasing sophistication in the way the nurses concerned were contemplating their care.

The RLT model does, however, offer some interesting insights that should not be overlooked, and could if developed, extend the applicability of the model to rehabilitation areas.

First, the model contains concepts that are particularly applicable to rehabilitation. Concepts such as a relativist definition of health, the impact of the environment on the independence of individuals, the importance of balance and dynamic equilibrium and its mechanism of maintenance, can all be seen to have relevance to rehabilitation nursing. Secondly, the interventions of the nurse as dictated by the model are particularly relevant to rehabilitation nursing. The nurse has to seek to prevent, solve, alleviate and teach the client to cope with, problems with activities of living. This perception of nursing contains some very important activities that are the central interventions of the rehabilitation nurse.

The question is, therefore, why is this model perceived as unsuitable for rehabilitation, as the experience of the stroke units would indicate? The answer lies in the concentration of practitioners on the physical aspects of the model identified in the activities of living. These activities mirror, to a great extent, the needs expounded by the Henderson model and are particularly useful in acute areas. The RLT model does, however, go beyond the activities of living per se and emphasies that each activity should be seen to contain three components: physiological, social and psychological. Concentration on the physical aspects of the activities is an outlook that misunderstands the model to the detriment of its wider use.

In addition to a broader understanding of the components of the activities of living, the model also identifies three other types of activities that broaden the range of actions undertaken by an individual in the pursuit of health. First are preventing activities, those that help avoid damaging features of the immediate environment. Secondly, the model identifies comforting activities, which are undertaken to provide the individual physical, psychological and social comfort. Lastly, and for rehabilitation nurses most significantly, the model identifies seeking activities, which identify activities such as the pursuit of knowledge, new experiences and the solutions to new situations and problems not encountered before. The possibilities of developing the use of the model along the lines of these activities, alongside the nursing intervention discussed above, would seem to open up the model to areas of supportive, educational and psychological care that have been accepted as lacking in its practical application.

The relationship between these activities and the activities of living is seen by Roper as a very close one (Roper, 1976). The significant feature of the preventing, comforting and seeking activities is that the use of these activities by the individual moves the model away from a purely functional interpretation, within which it is commonly entrenched. The criticisms of the model as being functional and solely concerned with the physical aspects of client care is therefore unwarranted, and the possibilities of the model given a broad interpretation of the definitions and fully encompassing all its levels of activities opens it up for wider and more considered usage.

Self-care

The concept of self-care is based on the belief that individuals will act in a manner that will maximise their health, by learning and performing activities which will support their health. Such a concept is now well established in the nursing literature as a central plank of the approach many nurses take to care, as a response to the passive recipient role perceived to have existed in earlier eras (Bennet, 1980). The fact that self-care and the resultant personal growth have assumed a perceptible position in health care is seen to be due to both the influence of consumer groups (Hickey, 1986) and the effects of the anti-professionalism of the 1960s (Norris, 1978). The importance of the concept is reiterated by the number of authors that have attempted to define it. Levin et al. (1976) defined the concept as a lay person functioning on their own behalf in the promotion of health, disease detection, prevention and treatment. This definition stresses the health maintenance and preventative strategies, whilst Hickey (1980) and Caley, et al. (1980) take a more life-long view that self-care is an individual's consistent improvement in their own health and wellbeing. This broader more life-long approach is conceptually extended by Brooke, Nyatanga and Walker (1986), Dean (1981), Orem (1985), and George (1986) to a definition of social proportions, in which self-care is a social phenomenon formed by complex societal conditions. These authors see these societal conditions as the relationship between man and the environment (Orem, 1985), families, groups and communities at large (George, 1986) and by Brooke et al. (1986) as a result of age, stage of inner development, sociocultural orientation and personal resources. However, the most cogent development of the concept of self-help is that developed by Orem in her self-care deficit theory of nursing; it is this approach that will be developed in this section.

Orem's self-care deficit theory of nursing

Orem's self-care deficit theory of nursing contains a number of concepts. These must be described before the theory's processes can be understood, and its implications for rehabilitation nursing explored. They are listed in Box 1.4.

Box 1.4
Concepts central to Orem's self-care theory

Self-care	In the drive for their survival, health, wellbeing and quality of life, adults learn to execute particular acts.
Self-care deficit	Where patients are unable to perform self-care due to health-derived or health-related limitations, then a need for nursing exists.
Self-care agency	The individual's ability to perform self-care will vary between individuals, dependent upon factors such as age, level of development, skills, knowledge and motivation.
Therapeutic self-care demand	This is the sum of the actions required by an individual to maintain health.
Nursing agency	This is the ability of a nurse to provide the care that is required to meet a client's therapeutic self-care demand.

These five concepts can be seen arranged pictorially in Figure 1.2, depicting the central relationships between them and hence the main thrust of the overall theory.

Figure 1.2 demonstrates that the basic relationships between the concepts is that in 'health', an individual's therapeutic self-care demands are satisfied by self-care through the individual's self-care agency. While this relationship is maintained, the status quo is preserved. When the situation arises in which the individual's self-care agency is no longer sufficient to maintain the required level of self-care (due to an altered therapeutic self-care demand or a

Figure 1.2
The relationship between the key concepts (reproduced with kind permission from Orem, 1991, p. 64)

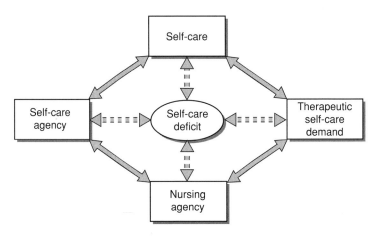

decreased ability on the part of the individual to undertake self-care) then an outside agent intervenes to deal with the self-care deficits.

Orem's theory and rehabilitation nursing

In relation to rehabilitation nursing, two aspects of Orem's theory will be discussed. The first of these relates to the problem of the delivery of self-care. A strong theme of normality as self-care delivery by the individual is seen to run throughout Orem's model (Aggleton and Chalmers 1986), with the emphasis on returning to maximal functional ability (Bowles, Oliver and Stanley, 1995) so as to regain individual self-care agency. Similarly, the focus on wholly compensatory care, as opposed to partially compensatory or supportive-educative care (Knust and Quarn 1983), so as to emphasise the transient nature of nursing interventions, should raise questions for the rehabilitation nurse. These problems, however, are not ones that should inhibit the use of Orem's model in a rehabilitation setting.

The first of these concerns the maintenance of self-care by the individual being perceived as 'normality'. A reading of the concepts defined above and depicted in Figure 1.2 does present a scenario in which the expectation is that the individual's self-care deficits are transitory, which by definition may not be the case in rehabilitation nursing. However, Orem does anticipate this problem by the introduction of the concept of dependant care. The concept of dependant care is the recognition that other individuals or groups can be aware of the existence of self-care deficits and can therefore be actively involved in care that seeks to ameliorate them. Orem gives four examples of this form of care, two of which are concerned with infancy and dependency: the family providing the care in the case of a child and the mother in the case of the new-born. The other two examples directly concern the remits of rehabilitation nursing, that is, the role of carers in the spheres of care of the elderly and of the disabled. The development of the dependant care concept is such that Orem's approach to self-care is augmented by the addition of the carer relationship that is central to the philosophy of rehabilitation. This relationship is illustrated in an expanded version of Figure 1.2 which can be seen in Figure 1.3.

Alongside the concept of dependant care is the associated one of dependant care agency, which is concerned with the ability of the carer to positively intervene and manage the dependant's self-care deficits. This once again is a central tenet of the philosophy of rehabilitation nursing, which is that a vital feature of the nurse's activity is to educate and prepare carers to deliver such care as they wish to and are able.

There is concern that Orem does not concentrate enough on the types of care that rehabilitation nurses undertake. Once again, a more detailed reading of Orem's writings indicates that this is not the

Figure 1.3
The relationship between the key concepts and the dependant-care agency (reproduced with kind permission from Orem, 1990)

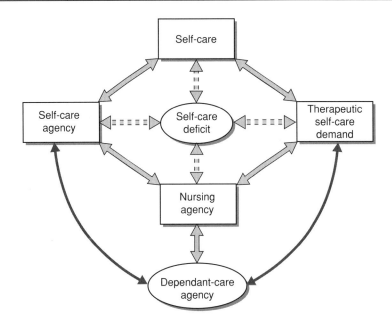

case. Orem describes nursing actions as 'methods of assisting' (Orem, 1991) and, in his commentary on Orem, Cavanagh describes them as the 'nature of nursing actions' (Cavanagh, 1991). Five are differentiated by both authors and can be seen as general ways of helping that can be used by one person so as to be of assistance to another. Orem emphasises that these methods of care may be initiated individually or simultaneously:

1. Acting or doing for another
2. Guiding another
3. Supporting another, physically or psychologically (the latter is best defined by the term 'understanding presence')
4. Providing for a developmental environment (which in essence implies that the nurse is responsible for the provision of an environment conducive to the client's recovery)
5. Teaching another.

The first three of Orem's methods of assisting can be seen as facilitative interventions, as the concepts of acting or doing, guiding or supporting, are clearly designed to facilitate the client's own actions in self-care. Facilitative interventions are interventions through which nurses expedite their care by actions such as 'supervising', 'encouraging', 'enabling', 'helping and boosting', and 'assisting'. What the methods of assisting do not cover are those activities that can be seen as non-interventionist, which seem to go beyond the remit of methods of assisting. Non-intervention covers those actions through which nurses temper or limit the extent of their interventions, such as 'intervening at the appropriate time', 'standing back', 'keeping hands off not hands on', 'giving them room', 'sitting on their hands'. The implications for care delivery are that these categories impose on the nurses' day-to-day actions a pattern of care that is focused on the client's contribution to their recovery, not the nurses'. The client's contribution is highlighted by the nurses' determination to limit their own input to the minimum required, while at the same time pushing forward the boundaries of the client's capabilities. Therefore, the methods of assisting as outlined by Orem represent only half of the picture. The addition of the concept of non-intervention completes the full picture of the nurses' actions in promoting self-care, not only in terms of the nurses' positive actions, but also in terms of how the nurses actually limit their interventions so as to promote the client's actions.

The concept of facilitative interventions is clearly laid out in terms of helping the client and is at the centre of Orem's theory of self-care. The concept of non-intervention involves decisions about when and how not to intervene. The nurse has to be aware of when to withdraw assistance, before the client is capable of undertaking care for themselves or with their caregiver. This inevitably involves risk-taking on a frequent basis. Non-intervention should be seen as extremely important to nurses involved in rehabilitation care, and as one of the defining characteristics not only of the way direct care is delivered, but also the way in which the whole of a client's care programme is approached.

Adaptation   The concept of adaptation is one which, unlike self-care, is in every-day usage. Adaptation as a general concept implies the ability to adapt oneself, or perhaps more importantly one's behaviour, in line with changing circumstances. However, even though this is a common-sense interpretation, two important criteria can be highlighted. First, adaptation is more than just physical change; the concept is concerned not only with physical but also social and psychological change, and as such, should be seen as a mechanism that effects the whole being of an individual. Secondly, given that change is inevitable, whether through natural development or through the traumas of every-day life, adaptation is a necessary process within the human condition. Given that change is a permanent feature of modern life, then adaptation should be seen as the normal state of an individual's situation. Within the sphere of 'normal' adaptation, the process is such a natural one, that is it generally unremarkable. However, given the advent of physical trauma or disability, the resultant physical, psychological and social impact on the individual may be beyond the capabilities of their own adaptive resources, and crisis results. Such an interpretation of adaptation, reflecting the advent of crisis, is the situation most frequently understood by health professionals as the meaning of adaptation in general. For example, Pollock (1986) defines adaptation not as a normal state but as 'the degree to which an individual adjusts psychologically, socially and physiologically to a long term illness; it may include psychological and social functioning as well as alterations in health status'. This formal identification of adaptation as a distinctive process does, however, predate Pollock. Helson (1964) describes an individual's innate ability to face and deal with change as their 'adaptive level'. The belief in the adaptive ability of individuals, and a belief that an individual is a dynamic system can be seen as the cornerstones for Sr. Callista Roy in the development of her Adaptation Model (RAM). The way Roy deals with the central concepts of the individual, the environment, health and the nature of nursing interventions are central to her model.

Roy (1984) describes individuals as being by nature, adaptive systems, constantly raising their ability to cope with alterations in their environmental stimuli. The need for nursing intervention arises when the degree of adaptation required by an individual is beyond the individual's present adaptive level, hence intervention is required to either raise the individual's adaptive level or to negate or ameliorate changes of environmental stimuli. For a clearer understanding of these relationships, some of the key concepts of Roy's model need further explanation.

Roy builds on the theory of an individual as a system and considers the individual as an holistic adaptive system. The term adaptive is taken to mean that, 'the human system has the capacity to adjust effectively to changes in the environment and, in turn, affect that environment' (Roy 1984). This stance is not new in terms of the understanding of the concept of adaptation, however Roy goes on to clarify the process by describing adaptive mechanisms and four major areas within which these coping mechanisms can be seen. These responses are seen by Roy to exist within the individual's adaptation level.

Coping mechanisms are seen by Roy to be the use of particular behaviours in response to environmental stimuli. Within the individual's every-day existence, such behaviours are required to deal with the normal variety of stimuli that the individual would expect to encounter. Coping mechanisms are also deployed to deal with the unexpected or the drastic, where the normal responses are insufficient to master the new situation and its stimuli. These forms of behaviour, whether routine or non-routine, are the product of normal development. Roy identifies two forms of coping mechanism that can be deployed regardless of the form of the stimuli; these are the regulator and cognator. The regulator coping mechanism is effective at a subconscious level and deals with physiological stimuli. The system is almost always the province of the autonomic nervous system and the endocrine system, and therefore automatic responses. The cognator coping mechanism is seen to be the conscious response on the emotional and judgemental level that addresses a psychosocial stimuli.

The concept of adaptive levels therefore describes the 'constantly changing point that represents the person's ability to cope with the changing environment in a positive manner' (Roy 1984). The adaptive level should be seen as a set of limits within which the individual is able to cope, based on their own developed coping mechanisms. Should the environment impose upon the individual stimuli that are above and beyond the adaptive level of the individual, then ineffective responses are to be anticipated, in the form of inappropriate or ineffective attempts to cope with that stimuli.

Henson (1964) also identified three classes of stimuli which Roy adopted for her model. The three classes of stimuli are focal, contextual and residual stimuli. Focal stimuli refer to those stimuli that directly impact upon the individual and necessitate a rapid response. Contextual stimuli are all other stimuli that can be identified as having an effect upon the response to the focal stimuli, and that are related to the focal stimuli to the extent that they may potentiate its effect. Residual stimuli are those stimuli that have an effect upon the individual which cannot be substantiated, i.e. the direct causal effect is not known but a relationship is possible. The identification of cause for a residual stimuli is important, as once a cause has been established, then the residual stimuli would become either focal or contextual dependent upon the nature of that causality.

Roy anticipates that all stimuli which affect the individual are the subject matter of the nurse's assessment, and should therefore be addressed on an individual basis. To aid the identification of the stimuli, Roy identified four adaptive modes to structure the nurse's approach. The four adaptive modes are the physiological mode, the self-concept mode, the interdependence mode and the role-function mode. The physiological mode deals with the five primary needs, oxygen, nutrition, elimination, activity and rest, and protection, which are generally the remit of the regulator mechanism. The remaining three modes are all psychological modes directly related to their titles, and as such are the remit of the cognator mechanism.

The relationship between these concepts is therefore as follows. The individual exists within an environment of stimuli, which is maintained in balance by the individual's adaptive level, which is the product of their regulator and cognator coping mechanisms. The system is kept in balance, given the continually changing environmental stimuli, by the individual's ability to develop their adaptive level over time, as developmental changes and maturity progress. There are, however, occasions when the individual's adaptive level is unable to cope with a stimuli. In this instance, it is the role of the nurse to identify both the nature of the stimuli that are affecting the individual, and that individual's adaptive modes with which support is required, until their own adaptive level rises to the stimuli or the stimuli is removed or dissipates.

The Roy model and rehabilitation

The Roy model has obvious strengths for the rehabilitation nurse. The basic concept of adaptation is one that is at the root of the philosophy of rehabilitation. The concentration within the adaptive modes upon the psychological as opposed to the physical needs also reflects the position of the rehabilitation nurse, who frequently encounters a client with a stable physical condition which may improve to a degree but will leave residual disabilities that need to be adjusted to. The model also identifies the importance of the patient and caregiver relationship within the mode of interdependence. This relationship, appreciated as central to the rehabilitation process, is fully addressed by the model and, along with the modes of self-concept and role function, has an obvious importance for rehabilitation nurses. Other aspects of the model are also directly applicable to rehabilitation nursing. The nature of the nurse's intervention is perceived as supportive, in that the nurse enables and enhances the individual's own coping mechanisms to deal with the stimuli, but also intervenes to alleviate the effects of such stimuli while this takes place. Similarly, the belief that the individual within a supportive environment (which includes both the carer and the nurse) is able to develop their adaptive level, and will rise to meet the challenge of the stimuli, is central to the positive approach required in the rehabilitation process. Central to this belief is the mode of self-concept.

Pertinent to any discussion of self-concept is the work of Rose Harvey (1992), in which she discusses the role of values in the adjustments required to be made by clients so as to successfully cope with their chronic illnesses. Harvey bases her work on the central idea that the values of physically injured or disabled people are the same as those of non-injured persons (Dembo, Leviton and Wright: 1956; Shontz, Fink and Hallenbeck, 1960). However, to adjust successfully to chronic illness or disability, the client must adjust these health values to a new view of health that is different to that which underpins the non-injured person's view of health.

These 'new' values are based on an enlarged scope of values which, for example, decreases the importance of appearance and contains the effects of disability. Such value changes can be seen as attempts to minimise the impact of disablements (Dembo, et al., 1956; Wright, 1960). The need is seen to be that the values used to define health must be altered to a different level, so that through a process of revaluation, an adjustment may be achieved (Dembo et al., 1956; Tornstram, 1975). The range of these values is laid out by Kristiansen (1985a; 1985b) and includes risk-taking, appearance, freedom and independence, as well as the value of health.

Concepts such as potential and adaptation are common as outcomes, and can be seen as an attempt to alter the client's beliefs so as to be in line with new value systems. A set of outcomes such as these, that are realistic and that do not have fixed objective endpoints can be seen to be reflective of the ideas laid out by Harvey. Outcomes such as 'returning home' and 'walking again' can be seen to be based on a set of values that are centred on a belief system grounded in the values of the able-bodied, in that they may not be realist, given disability. A differentiation is therefore identified which is logical given the situation of the majority of clients that enter hospital for rehabilitation, in that full recovery is not an option and adaptation to some degree to a new reality is essential for successful completion of that rehabilitation. The value of outcomes such as 'coming to terms with the new reality' and 'reaching their potential' seem to fit into the theoretical approach laid out by Harvey. Although this analysis points to a potential differentiation between outcomes such as 'returning home' and 'walking again', perhaps more commonly associated with the client's initial perspective, and 'coming to terms with the new reality' and 'reaching their potential', associated with the nurses' belief that the outcomes are set by the nurse with the clients and their carers, and are mutually acceptable, and form the basis of the client's care in the first instance. These potential differences are, of course, the result of the nurses' opinions, and the nurses' opinions of the clients' feelings, concerning the appropriateness of outcomes for clients and their caregivers. The use of the concept is operationalisation in Roy's model, in that it provides a systematic route for the nurse to address this potential differentiation and resolve it without undue concern to the client and with their consent.

Other concepts and theoretical frameworks

This section will briefly identify other theories and frameworks relevant to rehabilitation nursing.

Model of human occupation

(Keilhofner and Nichol, 1989; Kavanagh and Fares, 1995)

Based on systems theory, the model of human occupation is concerned with occupational behaviour which is defined as 'activity', in which individuals engage during most of their waking time. This includes activities that are playful, restful, serious and productive. The individual within this model is viewed as an adaptive being, interacting with the environment. Disruption caused by trauma, disease or illness will result in dysfunctional occupational behaviour by the individual.

Although this model is mainly an occupational therapy model, its focus on occupation makes it relevant to the concept of quality of life, and therefore may have useful elements for rehabilitation nursing practice.

Contingency model of long-term care

(Hymovich and Hagopian 1992)

The contingency model is drawn from a number of theories, for example, systems, adaptation and motivational theory, and provides a comprehensive framework for clients with chronic illness and disability. The primary focus is on family functioning and the health-care professional's role is identified as being to assist individuals and their families in adapting to the condition and its effects on their daily lives.

This model is comprehensive and has the potential to enable rehabilitation nurses to assess clients holistically, taking into account elements such as time, the community, coping, the individual and the family.

The illness-constellation model

Morse and Johnson, 1991

Based on adaptation theory, the illness-constellation model identifies illness as being an experience that affects the sick person and their significant others. The focus of the model is on achieving wellness within the social context, and it incorporates the experiences of individuals and families. The model can be seen as a process of adaptation and within it, different levels of adaptation are identified for both the client and their family.

This model enables nurses to identify the stages that the client and their family go through to achieve adaptation.

Health promotion models

(Ewles and Simnett, 1992)

Concepts related to health promotion which are pertinent to rehabilitation include illness, wellness and empowerment. Health promotion models include the education and the empowerment model. The relationship between rehabilitation and health promotion is discussed in detail in Chapter 9.

Maslow's hierarchy of needs

(Hoeman, 1996)

Maslow's hierarchy of needs, which is based on motivational theory, identifies the levels of needs which need to be met for an individual.

Role theory

(Hoeman, 1996)

Role theory identifies individuals as having a number of roles which make up their quality of life. Role theory can be identified as being the theoretical framework behind goal-planning which is discussed in Chapter 6.

Views of disability

The way rehabilitation nurses view disability has implications for their practice and their interactions with disabled people. It is important that nurses are aware of the different models of disability, and current legislation and its implications for practice. This section will briefly discuss different models of disability and highlight relevant publications which explore in more detail the issues surrounding disability and current legislation. The majority of these publications are written by disabled people.

Sally French, in her book *On Equal Terms* (French, 1994), identifies several disability models, summarised in Box 1.5.

Box 1.5
Disability models (French, 1994)

- Administrative models, which are often written into legislation and acts of parliament and which tend to relate to specific areas such as education and employment. These models are often rigid and dichotomous.
- The philanthropic (benevolent) model of disability, where disabled people are protrayed as being helpless, sad and in need of care and protection. Often a view taken by charities.
- Lay models of disability, which are influenced by other models presented by charities and the medical profession.
- The medical model of disability is based on the assumption that the problems and difficulties disabled people experience are a direct result of their impairment. Disability is viewed in terms of the disease process.
- The social model of disability identifies that it is society that disables, therefore there are no handicapped people only 'handicapping societies'. It is the failure of the social and physical environment to take account of disabled people's needs which cause them a problem. Disability is defined as 'the loss or limitation of opportunities that prevents people who have impairments from taking part in the normal life of the community on an equal level with others, due to physical and social barriers' (Swain, et al., 1994).

The most recent legislation regarding disability is the Disability Discrimination Act (1995) which seems to focus more on the medical model of disability than the social model. It is not possible in this book to go into more detail with regards to the views surrounding disability in this country, and the development of the disability movement. There are already some excellent texts available written by disabled people themselves. In Box 1.6 is just a sample which will challenge thought and promote discussion.

Box 6

Some views surrounding disability in the literature

- **Browne, S. E., Connors, D. & Stern N. (eds) (1985)** *With the Power of Each Breath: A Disabled Women's Anthology* **Pittsburgh: Cleiss Press**.
  A collection of poems and prose written by disabled women about their own experience of disability.
- **French, S. ed. (1994)** *On Equal Terms: Working with Disabled People* **London: Butterworth Heinemann**.
  Presents the social model of disability and addresses topics such as prejudice, the disabled role, images of disability and the disability movement.
- **Gooding, G. (1996)** Blackstone's Guide to the Disability Discrimination Act 1995 **London: Blackstone Press Ltd**.
  Provides a detailed explanation of the DDA and implications for disabled people.
- **Keith, L. (ed.) (1994)** *Mustn't Grumble* **London: The Women's Press**.
  A collection of poems and prose written by disabled women.
- **Oliver, M. (1990)** *The Politics of Disablement* **London: The Macmillan Press Ltd**.
  Explores the individualised and medicalised views of disability in relation to society and the political agenda.
- **Oliver, M. (1996)** *Understanding Disability* **London: Macmillan Press Ltd**.
  Explores issues such as the fundamental principles of disability, citizenship and community care, social policy, education, rehabilitation and the politics of the new social movements.
- **Swain, J., Finkelstein, V., French, S. & Oliver, M. (1993)** *Disabling Barriers – Enabling Environments* **London: Sage Publications**.
  This book challenges the notion that disability is either a medical condition or a personal tragedy. It is based on the experience of injustice and the growing identity of disabled people, and presents a new approach to the understanding of disability.

Conclusion

This chapter has explored the meaning of rehabilitation and the main concepts relevant to rehabilitation nursing. (Chapter 2 explores the history of rehabilitation in more detail). Although there are a number of meanings of rehabilitation, and a variety of definitions in the literature, the attributes of process, restoration, effectiveness, enabling, facilitation, learning and teaching are common to the majority of them.

Nurses have had difficulties identifying their role within rehabilitation, and one of the reasons for this is because of the complexity of rehabilitation, and the number of phenomena and concepts that are part of it. There are frameworks identified in the literature (this chapter has only examined a few) which can assist nurses in coming to grips with the notion of rehabilitation and disability and will enable them to give a high quality of rehabilitation care to clients. It is important to remember, however, that it is not always appropriate to adopt a model or framework in its entirety to a specific area of nursing practice. The place to start for nurses is perhaps to identify what their philosophy of care is for their clients, and then to choose elements from a number of models to create an eclectic model which suits their practice.

References

Aggleton, P. & Chalmers, H. (1986) *Nursing Models and the Nursing Process*. London: Macmillan Education.

Baldwin, S., Godfrey, C. & Propper, C. eds. (1990) *Quality of Life: Perspectives and Policies*. London and New York: Routledge.

Bennet, J. (1980) Foreword to a symposium on the self-care concept of Nursing. *Nursing Clinics of North America*, **15**.

Blackwell. (1994) Blackwell's Dictionary of Nursing. Oxford: Blackwell Seicentific Publications.

Bowles, L., Oliver, N. & Stanley, S. (1995) A Fresh approach. *Nursing Times*, **91**, 40–41.

Brooke, P., Nyatanga, L. & Walker, L. (1989) Facilitating the self-care concept using the experimental taxonomy. *Senior Nurse*, **9**, 8–9.

Brown, I. (1997) *Quality of Life for People with Disabilities*, 2nd edn. Chelterham: Stanley Thornes Ltd.

Caley, J., Dirksen, K., Angela, M. & Henrich, M. (1980) The Orem self-care nursing model. In *Conceptual Models of Nursing Practice*, eds. Reihl, J. & Roy, C. Newark: Appleton-Century-Crofts.

Cavanagh, S. (1991) *Orem's Model in Action*. London: The Macmillan Press.

Chipps, E., Clanin, N., & Campbell, V. (1992) *Neurological Disorders*. St. Louis: Mosby Year Book.

Cummins, R. (1997) Assessing quality of life. In *Quality of Life for People with Disabilities*, 2nd edn, ed. Brown, I. Cheltenham: Stanley Thornes Ltd.

Dean, K. (1981) Self-care responses to illness: a selected review. *Social Science and Medicine*, **15A**, 673–675.

Dembo, T., Leviton, G. & Wright, B. (1956) Adjustment to misfortune: a problem of social psychological rehabilitation. *Artificial Limbs*, **3**, 4–62.

Diamond, M. & Jones S. L. (1983) Ethics and the quality of life in chronic illness. In *Chronic Illness Across the Lifespan*, eds. Diamond, M. & Jones, S. L. Newark: Appleton-Century-Croft.

Draper, P. (1997) *Nursing Perspectives on Quality of Life*. London: Routledge.

Ewles, L. & Simnett, I. (1992) *Promoting Health: A Practical Guide* London: Scutari Press.

Felce, D. & Perry, J. (1997) Quality of life: the scope of the term and its breadth of measurement. In *Quality of Life for People with Disabilities*, 2nd edn, ed. Roy, R. I. Cheltenham: Stanley Thornes.

Fraley, A.M. (1992) *Nursing and the Disabled: Across the Lifespan*. Boston: Jones and Barttlett.

French, S. ed. (1994) *On Equal Terms: Working with Disabled People*. London: Butterworth Heinemann.

George, J. (1986) *Nursing Theories: The Base for Professional Practice*, 2nd edn. London: Prentice Hall.

Greenwood, R., Barnes, M.P., McMillan, T.M. & Ward, C.D. (1993) *Neurological Rehabilitation*. Edinburgh: Churchill Livingstone.

Harvey, R. (1992) The relationship of values to adjustment in illness: a model for nursing practice. *Journal of Advanced Nursing*, **17**, 467–472.

Helson, H. (1964) *Adaptation-level theory*. New York: Harper & Row.

Henderson, V. (1966) *The Nature of Nursing*. London: Collier Macmillian.

Hickey, T. (1980) Health and Aging. Monterey: Brooks/Cole.

Hickey, T. (1986) Health behaviour and self-care in late life: an introduction. In Self-care and Old Age, eds. Dean, K., Hickey, T. & Holstein, B. Dover: Croom Helm.

Hoeman, S. (1996) Rehabilitation Nursing: Process and Application, 2nd edn. St. Louis: Mosby.

Hymovich, D. P. & Hagopian, G. A. (1992) Chronic Illness in Children and Adults: A Psychological Approach. Philadelphia: WB Saunders Co.

Jackson, M. F. (1984) Geriatric rehabilitation on an acute care medical unit. Journal of Advanced Nursing, 9, 441–448.

Johnston, M. (1996) Models of disability. The Psychologist, 205–210.

Kavanagh, J. & Fares, J. (1995) Using the model of human occupation with homeless mentally ill clients. British Journal of Occupational Therapy, 58, 419–422.

Keilhofner, G. & Nichol, M. (1989) The model of human occupation: a developing conceptual tool for clinicians. British Journal of Occupational Therapy, 52, 210–214.

Kirkevold, M. (1997) The role of the nurse in the rehabilitation of acute stroke patients: Towards a unified theory. Advances in Nursing Science, 19, 55–64.

Kirstiansen, C. (1985a) Smoking, health behaviour, and values priorities. Addictive Behaviours, 10, 41–44.

Kirstiansen, C. (1985b) Smoking, health behaviour, and values: a replication, refinement, and extension. Addictive Behaviours, 10, 325–328.

Knust, S.J. & Quarn, J. M. (1983) Integration of self-care theory into rehabilitation nursing Rehabilitation Nursing, 8, 26.

Levin, L., Katz A., & Holst E. (1976) Self-Care: Lay Initiatives in Health. New York: Prodist.

Licht, S. (1968) Rehabilitation Medicine. Baltimore: Waverly Press.

Lippincott, J. P. (1985) The Clinical Practice of Neurological and Neurological Nursing, 2nd edn. Philadelphia: J. B. Lippincott Company.

McKenna, H. (1994) Nursing Theories and Quality of Care. Aldershot: Avebury.

McKenna, H. (1997) Nursing Theories and Models. London: Routledge.

Mason, T. & Chanley, M. (1990) Nursing models

in a special hospital: a critical analysis of efficacy. Journal of Advanced Nursing, 15, 667–673.

Morse, D. J. M. & Johnson, J. U. L. (1991) The Illness Experience: Dimensions of Suffering. London: Sage.

Norris, J., & Hachinski V. (1978) Intensive care management of stroke patients. Stroke, 7, 573–577.

Orem, D. (1985) Nursing – Concepts and Practice, 3rd edn. London: Prentice Hall.

Orem, R. (1991) Nursing: Concepts and Practice, 4th edn. New York: MacGraw-Hill.

O'Connor, S. E. (1993) Nursing and rehabilitation: the interventions of nurses' in stroke patient care. Journal of Clinical Nursing, 2, 29–34.

O'Connor, S. (1996) Stroke units: centres of nursing innovation. British Journal of Nursing, 5, 105–109.

O'Connor, S. E. (1997) An Investigation to Determine the Nature of Nursing Care in Stroke Units. Unpublished PhD Thesis. The University of Southampton.

Oxford Medical Companion (1994) Oxford: Oxford University Press.

Pollock, S. (1986) Human responses to chronic illness: physiologic and psychological adaptation. Nursing Research, 40, 144–149.

Preston, K. (1994) Rehabilitation nursing: a client-centred philosophy. American Journal of Nursing, Feb, 66–70.

Roper, N., Logan W. & Tierney A. (1976) The Elements of Nursing. Churchill Livingstone: Edinburgh.

Roper, N., Logan, W. & Tierney, A. (1990) The Elements of Nursing. Edinburgh: Churchill Livingstone.

Roy, C. (1984) Introduction to Nursing: an Adaptation Model, 2nd edn. New Jersey: Prentice Hall Inc.

Roy, C. (1990) Introduction to Nursing: an Adaptation Model, 3rd edn. New Jersey: Prentice Hall Inc.

Royal College of Nursing (1994) Standards of Care for Rehabilitation Nursing. London: Scutari Press.

Shontz, F., Fink, S. & Hallenbeck, C. (1960) Chronic physical illness as a threat. Archives of Physical Medicine and Rehabilitation, 41, 143–148.

Swain, J., Finkelstein, V., French, S. & Oliver, M. eds. (1993) *Disabling Barriers – Enabling Environments*. Milton Keynes: Open University Press.

Tornstram, L. (1975) Health and self-perception: a systems theoretical approach. *The Gerontologist*, **15**, 264–270.

Wade, D. T. (1990) Designing district disability services – the oxford experience. *Clinical Rehabilitation*, **4**, 147–158.

Waters, K. (1986) The role of the nurse in rehabilitation. *CARE-Science and Practice*, **5**, 17–21.

Waters, K. (1991) The role of the nurse in rehabilitation of elderly people in hospital. Unpublished PhD thesis. University of Manchester.

World Health Organisation. (1969) *International Classification of Impairments, Disabilities and Handicaps*. New York: WHO, Albany.

World Health Organisation (1980) *International Classification of Impairments, Disabilities and Handicaps* New York: WHO, Albany.

Wright, B. (1960) *Physical Disability. A Psychological Approach*. New York: Harper & Brothers.

Further reading

Akinsanya, J., Cox, G., Crouch, C. & Fletcher, L. (1994) *The Roy Adaptation Model in Action*. London: The Macmillan Press.

Cavanagh, S. (1991) *Orem's Model in Action*. London: The Macmillan Press.

Fraser, M. (1996) *Conceptual Nursing in Practice: A Research-based Approach*, 2nd edn. London: Chapman & Hall.

Hartweg, D. (1991) *Dorothea Orem: Self-care Deficit Theory*. London: Sage Publications.

Johnson Lutjens, L. (1991) *Calista Roy: An Adaptation Model*. London: Sage Publications.

McKenna, H. (1997) *Nursing Theories and Models*. London: Routledge.

Newton, C. (1991) The Roper-Logan-Tierney Model in Action. London: The Macmillan Press.

Roy, R. I. (1997) *Quality of Life for People with Disabilities*, 2nd edn. Cheltenham: Stanley Thornes

2 Setting the scene

June Bendall

Key issues
- The development of rehabilitation
- The development of different specialties
- Growth of specialised rehabilitation centres
- Attitudes towards rehabilitation

Introduction

The aim of this chapter is to give an overview of the history of rehabilitation. Exploring the past, by looking at the background of rehabilitation and how the different specialities have developed, will give a clearer picture of how and why rehabilitation has reached its present stage, and possibly, how the future may develop.

The development of rehabilitation

Society has always had sick and disabled people in its midst. Egyptian mummies have been found with evidence of arthritis, tuberculosis and club foot. The concept of rehabilitation dates from before the birth of Christ. Artificial limbs, surely one of the first aids to rehabilitation, have been found from approximately 100 BC (London Science Museum). Most early rehabilitation was concerned with getting people back to work. If this was not possible, they were usually cared for in an institution or by a religious order. Many of the early advances in limb fitting, for instance, were developed because soldiers needed to return to battle. Florence Nightingale, who is best remembered for her 'lady of the lamp' image, emphasised the importance of returning to work.

Rehabilitation and wars have always been linked together; wars inflict injury and injured people need rehabilitation. The Knights of St. John of Jerusalem founded hospitals and hospices in 1108 in order to nurse sick people, which included their fellow crusaders. One of the first centres was called the 300 Club, which was a castle where the Crusaders could recuperate (D'Arbon, 1980). The main reason for rehabilitating soldiers or knights was, of course, so they could fight again. As early as the 16th century, knights who lost an arm were fitted with a bronze artificial limb incorporating a hand with articulating joints which could hold a sword to enable them to return to battle (London Science Museum).

The religious orders, Monasteries in particular, showed concern for disabled people, who they cared for in hospices. The word hospice was derived from hospitality, meaning welcome, shelter and refreshment along life's journey. It was not until after the dissolution of the monasteries that the first English Poor Law was instituted in 1601. From then onwards, the care of sick, disabled, poor and homeless people became the responsibility of the local authority, which at that time was the Parish. Each Parish built and supported a workhouse, which was seen as a means of helping people to return to work, as well as the place where sick and disabled people could at least be housed, if not exactly looked after. Workhouses continued to be the answer in the UK until the early 20th century. However, the conditions in the workhouses were appalling. In 1890, a Bethnal Green workhouse was described as having 335 female inmates; 10 were blind, 26 were crippled, 100 were 'infirmed' and 65 were more than 80 years old, yet only one nurse was employed, whose title and function was the Labour Mistress (Smith, 1993).

In spite of reforms by philanthropists like Lord Shaftesbury in the late 19th century, the only solution for sick and disabled people was the workhouse. Florence Nightingale was concerned about the workhouses, and in letters written in 1864 and 1866, she refers to the workhouse reforms, saying that:

> 'the workhouse sick ought to have the best practical nursing, and a good wise Matron may save many of these from lifelong pauperism by first nursing them well, and then rousing them to exertion and helping them to employment'
>
> (Nightingale, 1989)

The emphasis once again was on returning to work. The founders of orthopaedic rehabilitation, Sir Robert Jones and Dame Agnes

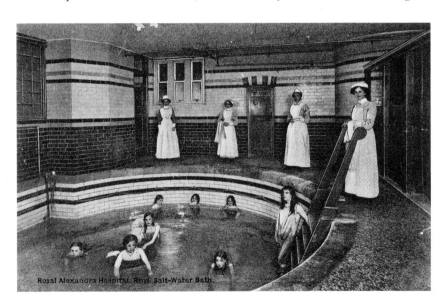

Figure 2.1
The Royal Alexander Hospital, Ryhl salt water bath – early hydrotherapy (1904) (reproduced with permission from Meadow books)

Hunt, were concerned with caring for their 'cripples', but finding them employment was also a priority (Hunt, 1938).

As society became more aware of the needs of sick and disabled people, the workhouses were no longer acceptable. Infirmaries were built alongside the workhouse, and later, specialist centres or hospitals were opened to cater for them (see Figure 2.1). Although returning to work is still considered an important part of rehabilitation nursing, we now put the emphasis on quality of life for our clients.

The development of different specialities

Each of the specialities developed at different times and at their own pace, but they all grew out of the need to provide rehabilitation. They were the beginnings of a needs-led service to a particular group of injured or ill patients. Sometimes it was government-led, as in the case of spinal injuries, but often it was to cater for increased numbers. More people were involved in accidents due to increased industry and road traffic. Increased medical knowledge helped more to survive. In the same way, people suffering from cerebral vascular accidents, elderly people and survivors of epidemics like poliomyelitis, also benefited from this increased medical knowledge. These people were often left with severe disabilities and needed rehabilitation. The emphasis was slowly shifting from returning to work, to restoring function, and leading as normal a life as possible.

Orthopaedic rehabilitation

Orthopaedic surgeons and nurses were the pioneers of rehabilitation services in the UK. In 1888, the construction of the Manchester Canal brought an increase in accidents to the area, and a local Orthopaedic Surgeon, called Robert Jones, set up first-aid stations and three base hospitals. This was the beginning of a concept that grew into an organised rehabilitation service (Glanville, 1977).

It was during the lifetime of Robert Jones that Dame Agnes Hunt showed an interest in rehabilitation. Her main interest was in orthopaedics, particularly in children. The main causes of children's deformity at that time was tuberculosis, osteomylitis and rickets. She realised that by treating them quickly and efficiently, further deformity was prevented.

Her family helped to open a convalescent home in Baschurch in 1890, and this became a 'home for cripples'. This was the beginning of the very first open-air orthopaedic hospital in the world. The cost per child was 8 shillings per week. There was no government grant available and this money had to be found by some charitable means, as most children could not pay for themselves. In 1902, with a total income of £415, the home dealt with 103 cases; 25 of these were 'cripples' requiring prolonged treatment (cripple was the description given to someone who was 'damaged, disabled or deficient'). At this time, society in general had no realisation of the magnitude of this crippled population, nor of its crying need. Some towns did have 'Cripples Guilds', and in London there was the Invalid Children's Aid Society, but much of the money gathered here was spent on splints. Unfortunately, as there was no one to supervise the application of these appliances, they were seldom worn, but greatly prized by the parents and often put on display on the mantelpiece (Hunt, 1938).

Apart from homes like Baschurch, there was no proper treatment, no aftercare, no hope for the future except for the workhouse. Sir Robert Jones, as he later became, was the Honorary Orthopaedic Consultant for Baschurch, and it was here that the famous Robert Jones and Dame Agnes Hunt partnership began. They shared an enthusiasm to improve the quality of life for 'cripples' in every way possible. In 1907, Dame Hunt decided that she would train nurses at Baschurch. The idea was that pupils came for 1 year and then would go on to 'proper training in hospitals', but some of them in fact stayed and were given the equivalent of an Orthopaedic Nursing Certificate (Hunt, 1938). The Orthopaedic Nursing Certificate was recognised in 1931. Robert Jones was involved with this training and is known to have said 'the orthopaedic nurse is here to stay' (Pearce, 1939).

During World War I, the home became a hospital for soldiers, with an increased number of beds – many housed in sheds and marquee tents – accommodating a case-mix consisting of 100 soldiers, 60 pensioners and 150 children. In 1921, it was reopened as the Salop Orthopaedic Hospital.

In 1927, Dame Agnes Hunt started a regular training centre to teach 'badly crippled' adolescents to earn their own living. Finding employment did improve their morale, as well as their financial situation. It is from this beginning that the Derwent Cripples Training College, the first of its kind, was begun (Hunt, 1938)

Following this example, other training colleges were opened. Queen Elizabeth Foundation for the Disabled was founded in 1934 as a residential training centre. The college set out to overcome the prejudice which existed so strongly against the employment of disabled people. Now there are eight centres providing information, training, assessment and rehabilitation. There are many other training centres throughout the UK, many of them providing a Disability Information Service.

Spinal injury rehabilitation

Although essentially still orthopaedics, spinal injuries have developed into a separate speciality and nurses have been trained in this field since the early 1950s. Ludwig Guttman was the pioneer of spinal injury rehabilitation.

Physicians have shown an interest in spinal injuries for centuries. Approximately 5000 years ago, an Egyptian physician described a complete lesion of the spine, adding the warning that it was an ailment 'not to be treated' (Guttman, 1976). In 400 BC, Hippocrates described paraplegia following a spinal lesion, mentioning the problems of constipation and dysuria, oedema of the lower limbs and bedsores. He advocated treatment of a large fluid intake and a special diet to help these clients (advice which has stood the test of time).

In the past, the vast majority of spinal injured patients did not survive the initial injury, but some attempts were made at spinal reduction. However, up until the 19th century, the main treatment of choice was conservative (Guttman, 1976).

It was World Wars I and II which swelled the numbers of patients requiring aftercare rehabilitation following spinal injury. Added to this, improved medical knowledge meant that more patients were now surviving the initial injury. Guttman realised that, in order to prevent these spinal units becoming 'a home for a clutch of doomed cripples', the provision of some sort of aftercare must be provided and that trained nursing staff was indispensable for this aftercare. With the increased number of spinal cord casualties, the UK government authorised Sir Guttman, as he later became, to set up a spinal injury unit at Stoke Mandeville. This opened in 1944, and it was here that the first principles of spinal rehabilitation nursing were practised. This still continues training nurses for spinal injury rehabilitation (Guttman, 1976).

Not all clients had the advantage of spinal injury rehabilitation. As late as 1955, clients were placed in boxes lined with sawdust to solve the problem of bowel or bladder incontinence (Martin, et al, 1981). In the 1960s, clients were often nursed on striker frames for years. Although things have certainly improved since then, nothing can replace the hands-on care of trained and experienced nurses (Strover, 1995). The life-expectancy of spine injured clients increased from 18 months in 1950 to 30 years or more in 1980.

In 1993–1995, over a third of spinal cord injuries were caused by road traffic accidents, just over a third by domestic or industrial accidents and one fifth by sports injuries (Grundy and Swan, 1995).

Poliomyelitis
rehabilitation

As sometimes happens, disasters lead to new developments. The epidemic of poliomyelitis was a means of establishing the importance of good nursing care combined with physiotherapy. It was an early example of a nurse/therapy-lead programme. These clients were usually treated in orthopaedic hospitals, and the orthopaedic nurse was expected to have a practical working knowledge of physiotherapy (Pearce, 1939).

Before 1960, poliomyelitis featured high in the disability classification. As a precaution against contracting the disease, one suggestion was 'to avoid other children between June and September' (Lewin, 1928).

The disease first became notifiable in the UK in 1912, and from then until 1947, the numbers varied from between 250 to 1600 patients each year. There was an epidemic in 1947, when numbers rose to 8000, and over the next 5 years, 20 000 people died or were very disabled by the disease. It was during the epidemic of poliomyelitis that the importance of positioning, as a means of preventing further deformity, was realised.

Sister Kenny was an Australian nurse who used hot moist packs in the acute stage, followed by passive exercises. This reduced spasm, but was thought to have no long-term effect on the paralysis (Breen, 1950).

The emergence of the vaccine in 1960 means the disease is now virtually non-existent in the UK (Nichols, 1971).

Head injury rehabilitation

Head injury rehabilitation is a relatively new speciality. As in other specialities, the number of people requiring rehabilitation following traumatic brain injury has increased through the effects of modern life styles, such as higher incidences of road traffic accidents, assault and sports injuries.

Man has sustained head injuries since biblical times, for example, in the story of David and Goliath. During the Crimean War, Mr. Guthrie stated:

> *'injuries to the head affecting the brain are difficult of distinction, doubtful in character, treacherous in their course, and for the most part fatal in their result.'*
>
> (MacLeod, 1858)

In 1855, 67 soldiers sustained head wounds penetrating the cranium – all were fatal (MacLeod, 1858).

Until recently, most head injury management meant little more than 'containment of the problem'. Finding an institutional niche was the only management these clients got, and they could expect to spend the rest of their days in an institution, which caused little inconvenience to others, and hopefully as much comfort as possible to themselves (Rose and Johnson, 1996).

The psychological problems of people with head injuries were, until recently, largely overlooked or unknown. Physicians often described these clients as neurotic compensation seekers. This interpretation of the profound problems, i.e. behavioural, cognitive and emotional, were common, and many clients were dismissed as unmotivated and irresponsible, and ended up in psychiatric institutions (Gronwall, Wrightson and Waddell, 1991).

World Wars I and II, together with the growth of the motor industry, increased the number of clients with head injury. Added to this, the ever improving medical knowledge and facilities meant that more people were surviving what was previously a fatal event. It was after World War I that neurosurgery became a separate speciality, and clients with head injury began to be rehabilitated (Boake, 1989).

Research was the main concern at this time, and the head injury centres at Oxford and Edinburgh gave priority to epilepsy and memory disorders. At Oxford, Richie Russell conducted a number of studies on the understanding and outcome of post-traumatic amnesia. It was later, during World War II, that neurosurgical centres were linked with rehabilitation centres. During World War II, a brain injury unit was established in Edinburgh. Here a psychologist called Zangwill became particularly interested in the psychological and social effects of head injury, particularly in the assessment of memory and the retraining of impaired ability (Boake, 1989). It was at Edinburgh that the use of psychology to form, or help in formulating, a general course of rehabilitation was first conceived. Zangwill argued that psychological rehabilitation, like all other forms of rehabilitation, should begin as early as possible (Zangwill, 1947).

40 years later, long-term management of the head injured continued to be a problem. The Royal College of Physicians Report on Physical Disability (RCP, 1986) said 'that in our experience head injury services are frequently not well organised, and there is considerable scope for improvement'. In fact, in 1986, Livingstone found that at 3, 6 and 12 months after severe head injury, between 75% and 84% of patients were receiving no rehabilitation services (Rose and Johnson, 1996).

The Medical Disabilities Report in 1988 pointed out that brain injury is 40 times more common than spinal injury and, though there is excellent National Health provision of special units for spinal injuries, at that time, there were no National Health rehabilitation units specially designed for individuals with traumatic brain injury. They were often left on surgical wards where no one was qualified to provide rehabilitation. In 1989, the British Psychological Society reported that the national UK picture of resources was dismal, with only 200 specialist brain injury beds in the whole of the country. As late as 1991, Wade highlighted the shortfall, stating that specialist services for the head injured are not available to most clients in the UK (Rose and Johnson, 1996).

Good quality acute care was available but this was not always followed up with rehabilitation. Now, as rehabilitation services are developing, the challenge is to promote the most effective outcome for these head injured clients, aiming at achieving stable and sustainable long-term outcomes, without unrealistic demands on health and social services. The primary problem in convincing health care professionals that rehabilitation is worth trying lies in lack of education about brain injury outcomes (Rose and Johnson, 1996).

There is evidence that early intervention with rehabilitation therapy does decrease the length of admission (Cope and Hall, 1982).

Once the client is ready for community re-entry, then local schemes are preferable. However, for the first few months after severe and moderate injuries, specialist units are necessary, both for the rehabilitation process itself, and also to act as centres of education, training and research (Barnes, 1995).

The Department of Health has given some priority to people with brain injury. 12 initiatives providing innovative forms of rehabilitation have recently been funded centrally. Researchers from Warwick University will evaluate this (DoH, 1996).

There has been a 15% fall in the number of head injuries since the compulsory use of seat belts. However, head injury is now the most common cause of death among young adults. In the UK every year, approximately 1 million people will receive treatment in an Accident & Emergency Department for mild to severe head injury, and of these, around 170 000 will have suffered some degree of brain damage (NHIA, 1995).

There is now good evidence of 'improved' survival following head injury compared with outcomes 10–20 years ago (Reilly, 1997; Feanside et al, 1993). However, more research is needed to see if the improvements in head injury care and rehabilitation can be translated into objective improvements in the quality of life for the survivors and their families (Reilly and Burlock, 1997).

Stroke rehabilitation

Stroke rehabilitation is often linked with care of the elderly, but although the incidence does increase with advancing years, strokes occur from childhood onwards.

Although stroke rehabilitation was not seen as a separate concept until recent times, disability due to stroke has been noted for centuries. Hippocrates wrote in approximately 400 BC about apoplexy, meaning to strike down, and said 'to cure vehement apoplexy is impossible and a weak one not very easy'. He noted that it occurred during the ages of 40 and 60 years, and especially during 'rainy weather'. He also wisely mentioned 'that it should be kept in mind that exercise strengthens and inactivity wastes'.

A thousand years later in 600 AD, Paul Agina coined the word hemiplegia. He also noted that in some patients, the power of speech is lost, and if it does not return in 14 days, the physician should try and do something about it (Bilik, 1937).

It was not until 1836 that right-sided hemiplegia was associated with loss of speech. It was 25 years after this, in 1861, that the word aphasia was used for the first time.

The first main reference to rehabilitation of stroke was in 1851 (Licht, 1973). In that year, Thomas Hung, Professor of Medicine in Albany, USA, retrained a 35-year-old blacksmith for loss of speech following stroke. He used various methods of reading, spelling and repeating words. In reporting his success, he gave credit to the wife of the client, who had performed most of the training. Exercising the paralysed limb was advocated to be beneficial during the middle of the last century. Robert Todd was a physician at Kings College Hospital in 1860 and spent much time studying and lecturing about hemiplegia, he wrote:

'I know of nothing which more decidedly benefits the paralysed limb than a regulated system of exercises, active when the patient is capable of it, passive if otherwise.'

(Licht, 1973)

The first hospital gymnasium is thought to have been in France in 1896, and was used for stroke clients. The physician concerned, Raymond, used the word rehabilitation and defined it as 'programmed gymnastics'. Although passively exercising the hemiplegic limb and encouraging the patient to walk continued to be advocated, there were some schools of thought who were concerned that it would lead to contractures, and until World War II, there were many faint-hearted physicians who endorsed great caution in applying early exercises.

Vascular surgery for stroke is relatively new. In 1951, the first surgical reconstruction of a carotid artery was performed (Licht, 1973).

There has been a steady growth in stroke units since 1953 (O'Connor, 1995), with most of them having a strong rehabilitation element. Clients under 65 years old are normally rehabilitated in neuro-rehabilitation centres. Every year, approximately 10 000 people under 65 will have a stroke (SA, 1995).

There is evidence that clients do better in a stroke unit. Mortality rates from 10 trials of specialised stroke units, in which clients were randomised between routine care on wards and admission to stroke units which included a multi-disciplinary team, showed a reduction in mortality of 28% in favour of stroke units (Langhorne et al, 1993).

It is estimated that 4% of the National Health Service budget is spent on cerebral vascular disease. Most general district hospitals have stroke rehabilitation units, both for inpatients, and outpatients, which may be well supported in the community. Returning clients to their normal environment, usually home, or back into the community, is one way of improving their quality of life. Therefore, community stroke rehabilitation teams are an important part of the plan for the 1990s, and many healthcare trusts do in fact have stroke rehabilitation teams which are based in the community.

The Health of the Nation document (DoH, 1992) targeted reduction in incidences of coronary heart disease and stroke as one of its five key objectives. This was to be achieved mainly by health promotion. However, improvement in rehabilitation was also mentioned which should 'aim to improve the quality as well as the quantity of life'.

The target is that by the year 2000, the death rate from stroke among people under 75 will be reduced by at least 40%.

No other single factor can contribute as much to diminishing the impact of disability as first-level prevention (WHO, 1981).

Elderly rehabilitation

Nurses have always been 'rehabilitating' elderly people as part of every-day nursing care, but this has only fairly recently been recognised as a speciality. Apart from the family, the care of dependent elderly people was originally the concern of the monasteries and then the workhouse and alms houses. The workhouses and the adjacent infirmaries catered for disabled, mentally ill, as well as old people. The health needs of older people who were unfortunate enough to have to enter such institutions were not considered separately. During Second World War II, a large number of elderly were transferred from hospitals to chronic sick wards or institutions, in order to make way for those with acute injuries being admitted from the war. Many of them stayed in these institutions until the beginning of the National Health Service in 1946.

Geriatric medicine began its life as a recognised speciality at that time. As the majority of clients came from workhouses, infirmaries or from chronic sick wards, little attempt had been made at rehabilitation, or even restoration of function. Pioneers of geriatric medicine recognised the importance of rehabilitation/early mobilisation, and nurses became actively involved with this, thereby helping these clients improve their quality of life. Many nurses had expertise in this field of nursing, and the nurses' model of management of these long-stay clients became the philosophy of care. There was a close liaison with orthopaedics and stroke clients in the early 1950s. Slowly, the rehabilitation of elderly people became a speciality in its own right (Andrews and Brocklehurst, 1987).

The multi-disciplinary approach was first used at the West Middlesex County Hospital in 1930, being thought to be a revolutionary process of client care (Barker, 1987). Now, almost all elderly care rehabilitation units use a multidisciplinary approach, often with the nurse as the coordinator.

There are now hospital-based care of the elderly units in virtually all healthcare trusts and most have a strong rehabilitation component.

Many of them are part of a stroke rehabilitation unit (O'Connor, 1995).

Rehabilitation services can be provided in a number of settings, in a client's own home, in hospital or in a residential home, and should recognise the longer period of time that elderly people may need (DoH, 1996)

Rehabilitation can be continued in the community which is the method of choice if at all possible. The Department of Health has funded a 3-year project relating to the elderly, examining hospital discharge and outcomes after 6 months.

The new Labour government has promised to provide 'a rational and fair framework for the services and support for the growing numbers of elderly people'. It is hoped this will include rehabilitation (Labour Party, 1997).

Amputee rehabilitation

This is not a new speciality for nurses. Like other forms of rehabilitation, nurses have been doing it for a long time, but this was not recognised and the emphasis was more on the acute nursing care of the amputee, rather than of the rehabilitation that followed.

As previously mentioned, artificial limbs have been around for a long time. Before the 20th century, the making and fitting of artificial limbs became a 'cottage' industry for those who could afford it. Many clients had 'homemade' peg legs. These were often beautifully made, and one leg, made of wood in 1884, was worn by the client from the age of 16 years until he died, aged 94. Some artificial arms were made for cosmetic reasons as a sleeve-filler. These were constructed from basket weave as early as 1900. However, some artificial arms were made to be functional. It is recorded that one arm was made for a lady pianist who played with this artificial arm at the Royal Albert Hall in 1906 (Queen Mary's Hospital Museum, Roehampton).

Before the discovery of anaesthesia, if the client survived the shock of the actual operation and the risk of post-operative infection, they normally coped well with or without an artificial limb. An early text book states 'the patient will learn to wear, adjust and use his appliance' (Pearce 1939)!

Industrial machinery, road traffic accidents and both World Wars have enhanced the need for limb-fitting centres, which include rehabilitation and walking schools. One of the first in the UK was at Roehampton. This originated in 1915 during World War I and was known as Queen Mary's Convalescent Auxiliary Hospital for Limbless Soldiers and Sailors.

Following World War I, limb-fitting centres were established throughout the country. By 1921, all these centres were brought under state control with staff becoming directly responsible to the Ministry of Pensions. This continued until 1953 when the Ministry of Health took over (English and Dean, 1980).

The role of the nurse in rehabilitating amputee clients is now well established. Counselling skills are very important, some clients are ill at the time of their amputation and need good nursing care and some need early rehabilitation before limb-fitting. Many clients are over 70 years old, so nurses need to have the skills to care for elderly people combined with amputee rehabilitation skills.

Cardiac rehabilitation

This is a new speciality but an increasing number of nurses are working in this field. Ischaemic heart disease remains the commonest cause of cardiac deaths in western societies, and the highest rates in the world are found in parts of the UK.

The first cardiac rehabilitation service in the UK was set up over 20 years ago, about the same time as coronary care units were opened. But, despite the large numbers of clients who might benefit, only a few have the facilities available to them. This is because there is a division of opinion amongst some cardiologists about the physical and psychological benefits of rehabilitation. As early as 1955, Gottheimer began giving cardiac rehabilitation to his clients in Israel, and a little later in 1957, in Cleveland, Ohio, Hellerstein and Ford produced guidelines for cardiac rehabilitation. Many of these have not been improved upon since.

Cardiac rehabilitation was established to stop clients becoming 'cardiac cripples' following myocardial infarction or coronary artery bypass. The clients and their relatives need reassurance and confidence to resume a 'normal' lifestyle. The purpose is threefold: teaching, support, and exercises in a safe environment. A nurse or physiotherapist is a likely person to coordinate the rehabilitation programme (Horgan, Bethell & Carson, 1992). Cardiac rehabilitation is not yet available to everyone. Fewer than half the health districts in the UK have established cardiac rehabilitation programmes (Chua and Lipkin, 1993).

Health of the Nation (DoH, 1992) targeted coronary heart disease by aiming to reduce the number of deaths in people under 65 years by at least 40%. As with stroke clients, the main objective was health promotion.

Growth of specialised rehabilitation centres

The rehabilitation centres were an important turning point, because for the first time, the government was looking at the needs of disabled people and at their rehabilitation. As with most early rehabilitation, specialist centres developed as a means of returning disabled people back to work.

In 1940, Mr M. J. MacDonald MP, said in the House of Commons:

'There is one aspect of the healing of the wounded, which I would like to mention, it is the secret of the maximum cure pos-

sible for the patient. It is a process known as rehabilitation. It is not sufficient that the wound may be healed, the wounded part of the patient must be enabled to function again, so that he may once more play his part as a worker. I have appointed an advisor on rehabilitation'.

(Oxford English Dictionary)

In 1941, there was a shortage of munition workers because everybody had been called up to serve in the forces, and for the very first time, the government became interested in the employment of disabled citizens. The Ministry of Labour and National Service introduced a scheme for training and resettlement. Arrangements were made to interview clients while they were still in hospital and training was arranged. During the war, over half a million disabled men and women were found work by the Ministry of Labour (Mattingly, 1981).

The first time the word rehabilitation was ever mentioned in the *Nursing Times* was on 19th January 1945, in an article entitled 'Rehabilitation of the worker suffering from nervous disorders'. This was followed by several other articles in the same year, but their focus was always on returning to work.

Thompson Committee 1941

One of the many committees that looked at rehabilitation·was the Thompson Committee in 1941. This was concerned with providing post-hospital rehabilitation. It was recommended that this should be the responsibility of the Ministry of Labour rather than the Ministry of Health. Other recommendations included a register of disabled persons at every Labour Exchange. This was a scheme under which employers with more than 20 workers must employ 3% registered disabled. Unlike the recommendations of many later committees, those of the Thompson Committee were promptly put into effect, including the 1944 Disabled Persons Act, which remained in force for over 30 years, preceding the National Health Service Act of 1946 (see Box 2.1).

As rehabilitation at this time was aimed at getting people back to work, employment rehabilitation, retraining and resettlement developed sooner and faster than medical rehabilitation.

It is interesting to note that the National Health Service Act of 1946 specified prevention, treatment and rehabilitation as its three principal elements.

Box 2.1
Acts of Parliament affecting the course of rehabilitation

1944 Disabled Persons (Employment) Act
1946 National Health Service Act
National Insurance Act
National Insurance (Industrial Injuries) Act

> **1948** National Assistance Act
> **1970** Chronically Sick and Disabled Persons Act
> **1973** Employment and Training Act
> **1996** The Disability Discrimination Bill

Piercy Committee (1953–1956)

This committee was set up to review the existing provisions for the rehabilitation, training and resettlement of disabled persons. Full regard had to be given to the need for the utmost economy in the government's contribution, as well as to make recommendations. It was actually this committee which recommended there should be centres for industrial rehabilitation or hospital rehabilitation centres, and that these should be planned carefully. It was not until 1968 that the first of these comprehensive centres at Garston Manor, Hertfordshire was opened. This committee expressed its concern about the medical professions' lack of interest in rehabilitation.

Tunbridge and Mair Committee (1968–1972)

These were set up to consider future rehabilitation services in the National Health Service. Their reports were unanimous in criticising the lack of information, coordination, effort and interest. The medical profession was once again criticised for ignorance and apathy.

The Mair Committee was much concerned with the need for medical leadership, and concluded that lack of interest in rehabilitation and failures in coordination could only be remedied by training specialists in rehabilitation. (It was not until 1990 that rehabilitation was recognised as a medical speciality in its own right.) It was during the time of the Mair report that the 1970 Chronically Sick and Disabled Persons Act was passed.

It was following this, in the early 1970s, that it was suggested that specialised regional demonstration centres were set up (see Figure 2.2). Some of these centres are still in existence today, and others have changed their purpose (Mattingly, 1981). In 1997, this is still the case; some have remained specialised rehabilitation centres, but many of them have closed or become outpatient centres, as getting back to work is no longer their main purpose. The specialised centres developed in response to the need for rehabilitation for that particular group of people at that time. Most severely injured clients will still need to be admitted to a specialised centre for head or spinal injuries. Stroke clients will do better admitted to a stroke unit. Other specialities may be able to rehabilitate in a unit which is part of a general ward, e.g. orthopaedics, care of the elderly. Amputee and cardiac rehabilitation may continue at day hospitals.

The specialised areas of rehabilitation continue to be centres of expertise. Many of them are now extending their rehabilitation into the community (see Figures 2.3 and 2.4).

Figure 2.2
Organisation of
rehabilitation in the
UK 1944–1981
(Mattingly, 1981)

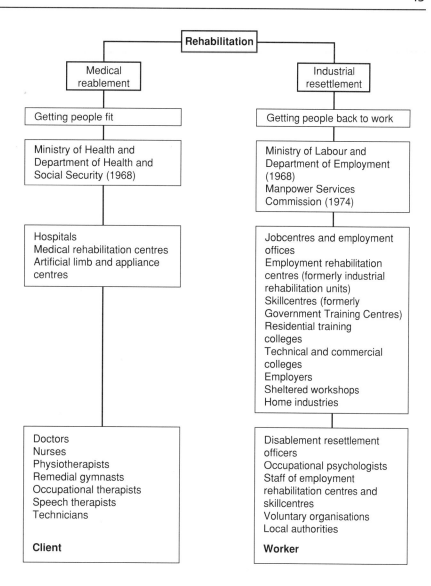

Attitudes
towards
rehabilitation

Exploring the attitudes of various professionals towards disability and rehabilitation, as well as that of society as a whole, gives us a clearer picture of how rehabilitation has reached its present stage. It may also help nurses be more aware of the problems facing clients once they have left the security of the hospital or specialised unit.

Attitudes to disability depend on the culture and era we live in, as well as the individual concerned. In Biblical times, disease and deformity was seen as a manifestation of sin – sins of the father being 'visited' on the children (Old Testament Exodus 34: 7). The disciples asked 'Who did sin? This man, or his parents, that he should be born blind' (New Testament St. John 1:2).

In the middle ages, disability was linked with evil. Shakespeare portrays Richard III (in Act I, Scene I) as twisted in body and mind:

Figure 2.3
Getting people back to work in 1954 (reproduced with kind permission of the Royal Star and Garter Home for Disabled Sailors, Soldiers and Airmen, Surrey)

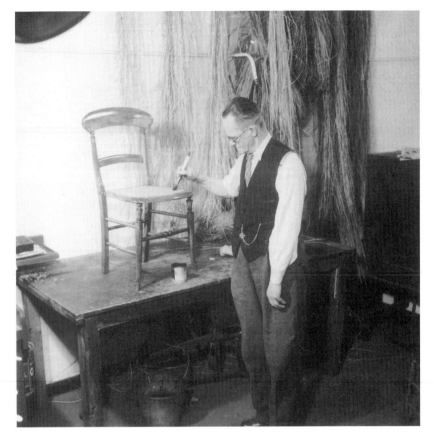

*'Cheated of feature by dissembling nature
Deformed, unfinished, sent before my time.'*

Although most early societies supported the sick, they often could not support long-term disabled people. The solution was sometimes a quick death. The Eskimoes placed disabled members of their society on free-flowing ice; the Indians placed poisonous snakes in their tents and the Greeks left them out overnight on a cold mountain. A quick death was seen to be preferable to a life of suffering (Martin et al, 1981).

Even now, in some African countries if a disabled person's judgement and memory are impaired (following a head injury for example), this is seen as shameful and they are treated as outcasts, whilst in some Arab States, if they are the head of the family, their position is upheld and they are treated with respect as head of the household.

In the USA, elderly people are expected to live alone, and guard their right to be independent very closely.

In Japan, it is the privilege of the elder son to have his mother or his elderly parents to live with him, and the daughter-in-law is expected to care for the aged. Frailty and illness are managed by retirement to bed. It was found in 1992 that 10% of the Japanese

Figure 2.4
Preparing for Exhibition Day, 1929 (reproduced with kind permission of the Royal Star and Garter Home for Disabled Sailors, Soldiers and Airmen, Surrey)

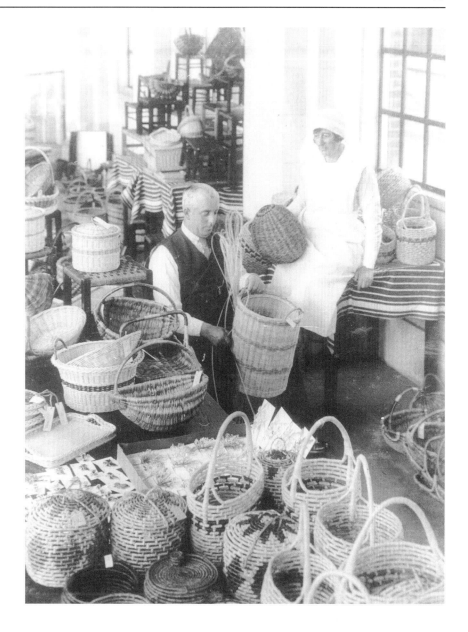

population over the age of 70 are in fact bed-bound. In Japan, it is impossible to travel in a wheelchair from the front door of the house to the toilet via the living room without transgressing important social rules (Walton, Barondess and Lock, 1994).

Until fairly recently, in Denmark, it was considered a matter of pride that disabled people were never seen on the streets. They were kept away from the 'sensitive' eyes of so-called normal people (Dambrough, 1980).

Most members of the public only become aware of the problems surrounding disability and handicap when the problems affect themselves or their family. People with physical disabilities are easy to recognise and are usually more acceptable than those who have invisible disabilities, e.g. cognitive and/or communication defects. Some people have taken to using a stick which they do not need, just to make others more aware of the fact that their speech defect or ataxic gait is due to brain damage and not drug or alcohol abuse.

Rachel Hurst, a disabled activist and the Chair of the Disabled Peoples International Group, was nominated for the United Kingdom Woman of Europe award for 1997. In order that she could attend the award ceremony a ramp was to be built, to replace an old unusable one; access was impossible without this. However, the day before the award ceremony, Rachel learned that payment had been vetoed for the ramp, so she would not be able to attend the ceremony unless she agreed to be carried up a number of steps in her electric wheelchair (an action which would have contravened European Union regulations on lifting and carrying). Rachel had been nominated for this award in recognition of her many years of work for disabled people's rights in Europe. This event happened before the United Kingdom Disability Discrimination Act, so the action was legal, if not acceptable (Hurst, 1997).

There are approximately 0.5 million wheelchair users in the UK but every-day places like cinemas, theatres, banks, car parks and toilets are not easily accessible to them, as any nurse who has taken a wheelchair person out shopping will have found.

Public transport

There are very few main bus routes adapted for wheelchairs, few inter-city coaches have this facility, and travelling in the guards' van on a train journey is still a common occurrence.

Accessible toilets on trains are rare. British Rail states all new trains will have 'them' but there would only be one per train. This could mean a long trip the length of the train for a disabled passenger (Barnes, 1994). Many hospitals are not wheelchair user friendly (Prince of Wales Advisory Trust, 1992).

Disability Discrimination Act 1995

The National Health Service is both employer of and major provider of services for disabled people, and nurses should be aware of the implications of the Disability Discrimination Act. One of the provisions includes the need to ensure that physical access is available.

Attitudes of medical students

Medical Students from St. George's Medical School spend 2 days at a neuro-rehabilitation centre during their neurological attachment. During this time, the students were asked about rehabilitation: what they thought rehabilitation meant, and how it affected client care. About 75% of the medical students had some idea of what it meant, but some thought of it as getting clients out of acute beds (which it does of course, but that is not the main objective).

Figure 2.5
'Restoring to working order' (reproduced with kind permission from the London Transport Museum, London)

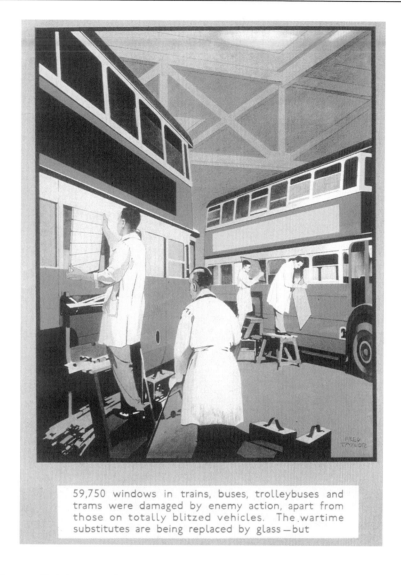

59,750 windows in trains, buses, trolleybuses and trams were damaged by enemy action, apart from those on totally blitzed vehicles. The wartime substitutes are being replaced by glass—but

Attitudes of nurses

Nurses finishing a degree course were asked about what rehabilitation means. Most of the nurses, about 80%, did have a good idea about the meaning of rehabilitation. However, several of the nurses said 'that units are often tucked away, rehabilitation for the elderly is in a separate unit'. These nurses saw rehabilitation as something that happens in a specialised centre or a specialist ward, and not something that they do every day. Some nurses thought that 'difficult' clients were sent to rehabilitation units. By this, they meant the clients that were difficult to handle in a ward situation (this is a shrewd observation as these patients are often referred very early). These nurses said that on the wards there is always a pressure to get things done, and actually taking time with clients or talking to them was 'frowned upon'. One student nurse felt that she was being observed, and to talk to clients is not considered to be one of her jobs. Many student nurses are not allocated to a rehabilitation setting during their 3-year training. However, numbers are increasing, mainly due to improvement in the staffing and status of rehabilitation units.

Encouraging clients to 'do things' for themselves is time consuming. Some nurses on general wards see rehabilitation as a low priority, and some found clients in need of rehabilitation on stroke wards as 'demanding' (Gibbon, 1991). Lack of intensive care beds is often in the news headlines, but lack of rehabilitation beds seldom makes the local newspapers.

The government's attitude

Governments have long paid lip-service to the concept of rehabilitation. As long ago as 1973, Sir Keith Joseph said:

> 'An improvement in rehabilitation standards can mean more to millions of people than almost any other medical advance.'

The last government passed a white paper in 1992 called Working with Patients. This had two objectives: to give clients, wherever they lived, better healthcare and greater choice of services available; and to produce greater satisfaction and rewards for National Health Service staff who successfully respond to local needs and preferences. This White Paper changed the funding arrangements, reputedly to give hospitals more control and make them self-governing. More consultants were employed to reduce waiting lists, general practitioners were given their own budgets. Whether this helped the cause of rehabilitation is difficult to say. This was followed by the Health of the Nation Document in 1992 which has been discussed elsewhere, as it targeted stroke patients and coronary heart disease.

Research and development in the Department of Health has funded some rehabilitation initiatives: (1) the twelve initiatives, providing rehabilitation for people with head injuries, which was mentioned earlier, (2) research relating to the elderly, examining hospital discharge and outcomes after 6 months, and (3) the European Community Helios Programme. This last programme aims to promote the integration and independence of disabled people by funding selective disability organisations to travel to meetings and conferences. There is also a multi-lingual database for disabled people as part of a separate evaluation programme, funded by The Department of Health (DoH, 1996).

The new Labour government priorities are: (1) to support the growing number of elderly people, (2) to change the annual contracts system (3) to put carers and users first (one of the examples that they use here is the fact that day centres are not open at the weekends and evenings when perhaps they are needed the most), (4) to improve community care, and (5) to produce a new patients' charter (Labour Party, 1997).

The Chronically Sick and Disabled Persons Act was introduced in 1970. On the second reading of this Bill, Alfred Morris MP said:

'If we could bequeath one precious gift to prosperity, I would choose a society where there is a genuine compassion for the very sick and disabled, where understanding is ostentatious and sincere, where if years cannot be added to the lives of the chronically sick at least life can be added to their years. Where the mobility of disabled people is restricted only by the bounds of technical progress and discovery. Where the handicapped have the fundamental right to participate in industry and society, according to their ability. Where socially preventable diseases are unknown, and where no man has cause to be ill at ease because of his disability.'

Alfred Morris MP, 1970

This was said nearly 30 years ago, but the society that Alfred Morris speaks of is not yet here.

Changing other peoples' attitudes is not easy. Some of the national associations like Headway or the Stroke Association have helped with good publicity and support. By encouraging clients to join these associations, nurses can help to prepare them for the world beyond the rehabilitation unit.

Conclusion

This chapter highlights that rehabilitation services have grown up in a very disorganised and haphazard manner. Up to the 20th century, disabled people were 'put away' in institutions supported by charity, and all rehabilitative measures were aimed at returning to work. The word 'rehabilitation' implied that the person had fallen from grace and needed to be reinstated. As the workhouses became unacceptable, hospitals and infirmaries catered for sick and disabled people.

Gradually, more people were surviving illness and injury and this, plus two world wars, and an industrialised UK, increased the incidences of accidents. Rehabilitation centres responded to the needs of these people, and the specialised centres grew and some became famous. Nurses changed their role from the labour mistress of the workhouse and the rather dictatorial nurses who told their clients exactly what to do (Pearce, 1939), to working *with* clients giving them choices and freedom to make decisions regarding the way of life best suited to them.

Although this chapter has looked at the history of rehabilitation in the UK, in the future we need to link with Europe and the USA in order to share knowledge, experiences and research.

Where do we go from here? Do we know what disabled people want? It has been suggested that rehabilitation is not only a product of institutional discrimination against disabled people, it is also a central component in the discriminatory process:

> 'It refers to a piecemeal welfare system of professionals and services, specifically designed to help disabled people learn how to cope with impossible social, financial, housing and environmental difficulties which would be totally unacceptable to any other section of the community.'

> 'In most cases the only part the disabled person is expected to play in the rehabilitation process is an inherently dependent one.'
>
> (Barnes, 1994)

It is hoped this is a minority view. The needs of disabled people in Derbyshire (Silbum, 1993) were listed by themselves and were:

- information
- housing
- technical aids
- counselling
- transport
- access
- personal assistance.

Residential solutions did not play a part.

Most rehabilitation nurses are working with people who have acquired a brain injury or spinal cord injury fairly recently. These people are learning to live with their disability and need rehabilitation. People who have been disabled for some time have usually acquired rehabilitation skills and are looking towards a society and environment that does not restrict them. They wish (quite rightly) to live in the community with as much 'freedom' as possible. This is often denied them (Barnes, 1994).

More rehabilitation services are now being set up in the community. Many specialised centres have their own outreach facilities. Spinal units have had good follow-up services for years. Very careful discharge planning from the specialised units into the community is one of the best ways to integrate the disabled person back into a familiar community setting. The new Labour government policy promises to improve community care, saying 'at worst it can mean neglect, dreadful loneliness and degrees of stress that destroys families, at best it can enhance the quality of life through autonomy, independence and a sense of personal dignity' (Labor Party, 1997).

History has taught us that making society aware of the needs of the disabled and aware of the need for rehabilitation will help to change the outlook of both society and the government. Putting people back into the community means that we are more aware, watching someone in a wheelchair, having to bump up and down the pavement or denied access into the bank, for example, or watching the delight in a child's face when their wheelchair is able to be accepted on an ordinary bus, helps us be more aware of what can be achieved.

Rehabilitation nurses can work with clients in general hospitals, in specialised units and in the community. Most clients following a brain injury or a spinal injury will need rehabilitation in all these settings. Along with the orthopaedic nurse of 90 years, the rehabilitation nurse is here to stay.

Rehabilitation is an endless search for possibilities, while learning to accept that limitations of body, mind, money, time, architecture, and society are real. It means the recognition and acknowledgement of one's own limitations without shame. It is aiming toward independence, but identifying areas where dependence is appropriate and necessary. It is fostering an atmosphere of trust and understanding between the dependent and the depended upon (Dittmar, 1989).

Questions for discussion	■ Where should rehabilitation take place? ■ Have we learnt any lessons from the past? ■ What is the future for rehabilitation in this country? ■ As professionals, are we doing enough to change attitudes towards disability and rehabilitation?

References

Andrews, K. & Brocklehurst, J. (1987) *British Geriatric Medicine in the 1980s.* London: King's Fund.

Barker, W. (1987) *Adding Life to Years.* Baltimore: The John Hopkins University Press.

Barnes, C. (1994) *Disabled People in Britain.* London: Hurst & Co.

Barnes, M. (1995) *A Regional Service for Traumatic Brain Injury Rehabilitation.* London: Chapman and Hall.

Bilik, S.E. (1937) Treatment of hemiplegia. *Archives of Physical Therapy,* **18**, 495.

Boake, C. (1989) A history of cognitive rehabilitation of head injury patients 1915–1980. *Journal of Head Trauma Rehabilitation,* **4**, 1–8.

Breen G. (1950) *Fever Nursing.* Edinburgh: E.S. Livingstone Ltd.

British Psychological Society (1989) *Services for Young Adults with Acquired Brain* Damage. Working Party Report. Leicester: British Psychological Society.

Chua, T.P. & Lipkin, D (1993) Cardiac Rehabilitation. *British Medical Journal,* **306**, 731–732.

Cope, O.N. & Hall, K.N. (1982) Head injury rehabilitation. *Physical Medicine and Rehabilitation,* **63**, 433–437.

Dambrough, A. (1980) Miracles for the many. (Report of the World Congress of Rehabilitation.) *Nursing Mirror,* **151**, 28–29.

D'Arbon, P. (1980) Rehabilitation yesterday and today. *The Lamp,* **37**, 16–18.

Department of Health (1992) *Health of the Nation.* London: HMSO.

Department of Health (1996) *Research and Development.* London: HMSO.

Dittmar, S. (1989) *Rehabilitation Nursing,* pp. 8–9. St Louis: Mosby.

English, A. & Dean, A. (1980) *The Artificial Limb Service Booklet.* Roehampton: DHSS Limb Fitting Centre.

Gibbon, B. (1991) A reassessment of nurses attitude towards stroke patients in general medical wards. *Journal of Advanced Nursing,* **16**, 1336–1342.

Glanville, H.J. (1977) What is rehabilitation: an inaugural lecture. *Rehabilitation*, **100**, 13–25.

Gronwall, D. Wrightson, P. & Waddell, P. (1991) *Head Injury – The Facts.* Oxford: Oxford University Press.

Grundy, D. & Swan, A. (1995) *ABC of Spinal Cord Injury.* London: British Medical Journal.

Guttman, L. (1976) *Spinal Cord Injuries.* Oxford: Blackwell Scientific Publications.

Horgan, J., Bethell, H. & Carson, P. et al. (1992) British Heart Foundation Working Party report on cardiac rehabilitation. *British Heart Journal*, **67**, 412–418.

Hunt, A. (1938) *This Is My Life.* London: Blackie & Son.

Hurst, R. (1996) Disabled Europeans Euro Update. *Journal of Disabled Peoples International*, 5.

Labour Party (1997) *Renewing the NHS.* London: Labour Party.

Langhorne, P., Williams B., Gilchrist, W., et al. (1993) Do stroke units save lives. *The Lancet*, **342**, 395–398.

Lewin, I. (1928) *Orthopaedic Surgery for Nurses*, p. 57. Philadelphia: W. B. Saunders & Co.

Licht, S. (1973) Stroke, a history of its rehabilitation: Walter J. Zeiter lecture. *Archives of Physical and Medical Rehabilitation*, **54**, 10–17.

MacLeod, C. (1858) *Notes on the Surgery of War in the Crimea,* p. 175. Edinburgh: John Churchill.

Martin, M., Holt, N.B. & Hicks, D. (1981) *Comprehensive Rehabilitation Nursing.* New York: McGraw Hill.

Mattingly, S. (1981) *Rehabilitation Today in Great Britain.* London: Update Books.

Medical Disability Society (1988) *The Management of Traumatic Brain Injury.* London: The Medical Disability Society.

National Head Injuries Association (1995) *Headway.* Nottingham: National Head Injuries Association Ltd.

Nichols, P. (1971) *Rehabilitation of the Severely Disabled.* London: Butterworth Press.

Nightingale, F. (1989) *Ever Yours, Florence Nightingale Selected Letters*, p. 246. London: Virago Press.

O'Connor, S. (1995) Results of a survey of stroke units in the English regions in the NHS. *British Journal of Therapy and Rehabilitation*, **2**, 435–440.

Oxford English Dictionary *Rehabilitation* xiii, 2nd edn. Oxford: Clarendon Press.

Pearce, E. (1939) *Orthopaedic Nursing*, pp. 5, 615. London: Faber and Faber.

Prince of Wales Advisory Trust (1992) *A Charter for Disabled People Using Hospitals.* London: The Royal College of Physicians.

Reilly, P. & Burlock, R (1997) *Head Injury. Pathophysiology and Management of Severe Head Injury.* London: Chapman Hall Medical.

Rose, D. & Johnson, D. (1996) In *Brain Injury and After: Towards Improved Outcomes.* Chichester: J. Wiley & Sons.

Rowe, F. (1945) Rehabilitation of the worker suffering from nervous disorders: role of the nurse. *Nursing Times*, **XLI**, 34.

Royal College of Physicians (1986) Physical Disability in 1986 and Beyond. *Journal of Royal College of Physicians*, **20**, 30–37.

Silbum, L. (1993) *Disabling Barriers Enabling Environments*, p. 219. London. Sage Publications.

Smith, F. B. (1990) *The People's Health 1830–1910*, p. 387. London: Weidenfeld & Nicholson.

Stroke Association (1995) London: Stroke Association, associated with the Chest, Heart and Stroke Association.

Strover, G. (1995) Review of 40 years of rehabilitation issues in spinal cord injury. *Journal of Spinal Cord Injury*, **18**, 175–182.

Walton, J., Barondess, J. & Lock, S. (1994) *Oxford Medical Companion.* Oxford: Oxford University Press.

World Health Organisation (1980) *A Manual of Classification Relating to the Consequence of Disease.* Geneva: WHO.

Zangwill (1947) Psychological aspects of rehabilitation in cases of brain injury. *British Journal of Psychology*, **37**, 60–69.

Further reading

Hunt, A. (1938) *This is My Life.* London: Blackie & Son.

This is an autobiography of Agnes Hunt.

Glanville, H.J. (1977) What is rehabilitation: an inaugural lecture. *Rehabilitation*, **100**, 13–25.

Nightingale, F. *Ever Yours.* London: Virago Press.

3 The team

Hilary Whitelock

Key issues

- The rehabilitation team
- Multidisciplinary teams
- Interdisciplinary teams
- Transdisciplinary teams
- Roles of team members
- Team building
- Goal setting

Introduction

There is widespread agreement that the rehabilitation team is central to the successful management of clients with disability. Rehabilitation is a complex subject or group of subjects, making it unlikely that any one discipline could cover all the areas of treatment required by this client group. It is for these reasons that this chapter considers teamwork and the structure and function of a team, particularly a successful team. It then considers three approaches to forming teams used in the rehabilitation setting: multidisciplinary, interdisciplinary and transdisciplinary. Concepts within teamwork, such as the keyworker role, team building and goal setting are introduced. The roles of various team members are outlined.

Effective teamwork is not always easy to achieve, team members need to understand each other's roles and realise the areas of overlap to ensure a coordinated and collaborative approach. The client is often confused by the different professionals' contributions and it is essential to spend time in explaining the benefits of the team approach.

Team building is vital to prepare professionals for the demands of teamworking. Given that problems of communication, coordination of effort, and role overlap, amongst others, do actually arise in practice, it is crucial that team members are supported, trained and supportive of each other within the team setting. Teams that have supportive structures in place, like interdisciplinary case notes, integrated care pathways, performance appraisal, operational policies and joint action plans, can rely on these to make their contributions as meaningful and effective as possible.

The rehabilitation team

The rehabilitation team is a group of professionals who work together to achieve a goal or goals which have been set. The team aims to provide quality care to the client. According to Shirley Embling (1995), the Concise Oxford Dictionary defines teamwork as, 'a combined effort or organised cooperation'. Blake and Mouton (1964), as cited by Embling (1995), provide an illustrative definition, stating that the word 'team' refers to any set of individuals who co-operate in accomplishing a single overall result. The salient features of an effective team are clearly provided by Embling (1995), as she advocates their necessity to accomplish effective teamwork (see Box 3.1).

Box 3.1
Important features of an effective team

- Shared Goals
- Interdependence
- Cooperation
- Coordination of activities
- Task specialisation
- Division of effort
- Mutual respect

(Embling, 1995)

Illustrative definitions are further explored by Wood (1993), who advises that many definitions of teamwork are available, e.g., Brill (1976), Furnell et al. (1987) and Dingwall (1980). They should, however, be viewed with caution and from a critical perspective, as theory does not always reflect the reality of the particular situation.

What makes a successful team?

There are many attributes to a successful and effective team. This is often termed a commitment team, or performing team. Such teams are perceived to add value to the service they exist within, and are described as synergistic (Eales-White, 1996). There are many factors that can contribute to the successful performance of the team, some of which are listed in Box 3.2.

Box 3.2
Factors contributing to successful team performance

- Clear objectives within the team
- Sound procedures for decision-making
- Members support each other with a high degree of trust between them
- Appropriate skill mix
- Even workload
- Members understanding of each other's roles
- Cooperation
- Ability to learn from mistakes
- Focus on problem solving
- Flexibility, honesty and openness
- Regular meetings to discuss ways of improving team performance, and to review operational goals, purpose and direction

- Highly skilled leadership
- Confrontation of issues and conflicts in an open way
- Commitment and involvement
- Enthusiasm, energy and fun
- Good communication, questioning and listening skills

Focusing on the team's strengths is particularly useful, building on the individual member's strengths is critical, and it is crucial to the successful performance of the team that its members are involved at all times in the problem-solving and decision-making processes.

Structure and function of the team

The main function of the team is to provide an efficient service to clients. In rehabilitation, there tends to be focus on function and functional improvement, and therefore on functional outcomes. It follows then, that the aims of the team address these areas. The way the team sets out to achieve these outcomes is certainly important and, according to Bakheit (1996), there are several prerequisites for effective functioning of a rehabilitation team. Bakheit explains that the objective of the team is to deliver a high standard of care that is tailored to the client's needs. He lists the features in Box 3.3 as necessary for effective team function.

Box 3.3
Necessary features for effective team functioning

- A balanced team structure
- A competent leader
- A clear operational policy
- Process of team activity
- A decision-making method
- Clear channels of communication
- Clearly defined roles, responsibility and accountability of individual team members

(Bakheit, 1996)

The reasons for these features being considered as critical in determining improved client outcome are unclear. But if the functioning of the team is based on clear operational guidelines, then its members are free to practice more confidently within these boundaries, thus forming a strong foundation for delivery of care. The argument in favour of interdisciplinary teams providing the client with a better service than they would have otherwise received from an individual profession is proposed and should be acted upon (Ovretveit, 1986).

The structure or composition of a team varies considerably from setting to setting. It is largely dependent on the client group served and is also affected by the resources available. In most instances, there is likely to be a central group of professional team members. These are complimented by a peripheral group that joins the team as and when necessary, or as agreed on a regular basis. These peripheral members play a supportive, advisory and specialist role. The central team usually consists of rehabilitation nurses, the rehabilitation physician, a physiotherapist, an occupational therapist, a speech and language therapist, a psychologist and a social worker. The peripheral members include dieticians, chiropodists, other specialist doctors, prosthetists, rehabilitation engineers, pharmacists, recreational therapists, community care professionals and in some cases members from the voluntary agencies.

The clients and their relatives are considered an integral part of the team (see Figure 3.1). Without partnership, teamwork aims and function become meaningless in the rehabilitation setting. Roles of the team members, including that of the client and family members, will be looked at later in this chapter.

Before we go on to look at the different approaches used in the rehabilitation setting, bear in mind that it is widely accepted that the team approach is considered to be the the model of choice in rehabilitation today (Bakheit, 1996). Bakheit believes that it is important to maximise the potential benefits of teams to achieve better outcomes of treatment. But he also points out that the advantages of teamwork are still disputed and advocates further studies in this field.

Three team approaches are seen in the rehabilitation setting: multidisciplinary, interdisciplinary and transdisciplinary. They differ conceptually and are briefly introduced below.

Figure 3.1
A rehabilitation team – the client and family are seen as an integral part of the team

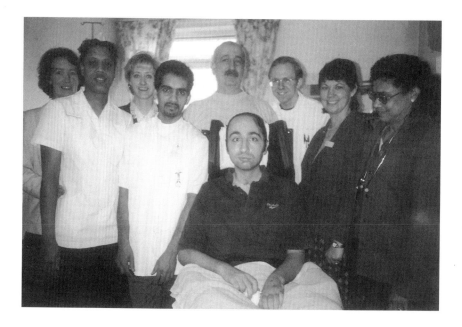

Multi-disciplinary teams

The multidisciplinary approach is characterised by several factors:

- Each discipline within the team works towards discipline-related goals.
- Team members work within the boundaries of their profession.
- Progress is discussed formally at team meetings.
- Effective communication is considered vital.
- The client's role is minimal.

On admission, as an inpatient, as a day case or within a multidisciplinary assessment clinic (where this facility exists), the client is initially assessed by all the members of the team separately. They then meet, usually without the client being present, to discuss problems identified, management, and planned sessions of therapy. Review and evaluation takes place at regular meetings, and at more formal case conferences, when the client and carers are involved.

Comprehensive assessment of patients with severe and complex physical and psychological disabilities is made possible by the multidisciplinary team using a collective problem-solving approach. Some areas have set up multidisciplinary day assessment clinics, to enable referrals and assessments to be carried out. Areas which employ this model aim to provide the patient with a coordinated service on one visit, when more time can be devoted to specific needs and advice can be given based upon the assessments of the team as a whole. This helps reduce the number of visits a patient has to make as they will see a nurse, a rehabilitation physician, an occupational therapist, a physiotherapist, a speech therapist, as well as a psychologist and a dietician.

Certain considerations within the concept of the multidisciplinary team need to be addressed further. First, the concept is well accepted today and is widely used in different settings, although it has been suggested by Shirley Embling (1995), that the concept of multidisciplinary teamwork is not always fully understood by many health care workers. Secondly, team members often have little understanding of each other's roles. And finally, it has been stated by Muir Giles and Clark-Wilson (1993) that the effective coordination of clients' care is difficult to achieve.

Inter-disciplinary teams

Interdisciplinary team work is considered the most suitable approach upon which to base activity in the post-acute rehabilitation setting (Pfieffer, 1980; Muir-Giles and Clark-Wilson, 1993). The main features of the interdisciplinary team are goal directedness, disciplinary articulation, communication, flexibility, and conflict resolution (Mandy, 1996).

This approach firstly allows for overall coordination of goals. The team usually meets the client, and then jointly, i.e. with each other and the client, assess the problems and agree on management goals.

The process involves the client closely, and the team members apply their joint skills to each problem or goal. Planned review takes place, usually at regular team meetings and in the form of goal-planning sessions and case conferences, where the client and relatives are involved.

This approach is obviously beneficial, as many goals do not always fit neatly into specific disciplinary domains. Examples of this can been seen in practice, for instance, in a client with poor posture and positioning, where these can adversely affect a swallowing problem. This is a common scenario encountered in individuals suffering from multiple sclerosis or motor neurone disease. The speech therapist works alongside occupational therapists, nurses and carers to ensure optimal swallowing, in a good position, whilst achieving adequate nutrition; there is opportunity for teaching input from all disciplines to achieve the overall goal. They intervene, cross invisible disciplinary boundaries and respond to the client's needs in the true context of interdisciplinary teamwork.

This approach is, however, sometimes considered very stressful for individual therapists, who are used to treating patients with a traditional approach. It is also very time-consuming as coordination necessarily takes up many professionals' time. Interdisciplinary teamwork relies on flexibility of the individual team members. It also relies on increasing understanding of each others' roles, as without this, conflict can occur when boundaries are crossed.

Petrie (1976) refers to the concept of 'cognitive mapping', which suggests that different disciplines use different concepts, modes of enquiry, problem definition and general ideas of what makes up each discipline. One example of this is where new staff are joining the team, and do not know other team members' cognitive maps, and need organised induction to enable them to understand and feel a part of the team. Team members need to take account of these facts to avoid common misunderstandings.

Mandy (1996) suggests that the key to avoiding conflicts in interdisciplinary teamwork is to introduce effective common training and education (see Box 3.4). He states that evidence from abroad shows that in such areas where this takes place, interprofessional understanding and collaboration increase, thus increasing the effectiveness of the approach.

Box 3.4
Key points of inter-disciplinary teams

> - Interdisciplinary care is a more appropriate nomenclature than multidisciplinary care.
> - Barriers to interdisciplinary teamwork must be overcome.
> - The key to overcoming those barriers is integrated undergraduate education.
>
> (Mandy, 1996)

Trans-disciplinary teams

The transdisciplinary team approach has recently been well described by Jackson and Davies (1995). They give us a clear definition, in relation to their work at the Transitional Rehabilitation Unit (TRU) in Wigan. They reflect that there is no other clear definition available, and have based their approach on the work of Leland et al. (1988) and Sachs (1991), who were also working in the fields of brain injury rehabilitation. Their work is seen as of considerable importance as it translates the theory of transdisciplinary teams into a practical working approach. Figure 3.2 shows the schematic representation of the transdisciplinary team used at the TRU in Wigan (Jackson and Davies, 1995).

This approach is highly organised and consists of rehabilitation professionals and non-professionals who are designated specific roles within the organisation: case organisers, clinical team, primary rehabilitation coach, and coaching teams. Case organisers are responsible for the client's rehabilitation programme. They are experts, professionally qualified and experienced. They have designated clients and are responsible for the direct communication and intervention with the client and family. The role of the clinical team is to develop service strategy, to train staff, and to address quality-assurance issues. They also fulfil a supervisory, expert consultant role. The primary rehabilitation coach is an internally-trained non-professional who is responsible for carrying out the hands-on therapy programme. They work with the case organisers in an effort to solve problems, and in setting and reaching of goals. The coaching teams provide back-up for the primary rehabilitation coaches and are designated specific clients, and give any support required by these clients.

This approach offers consistency, effective use of expert resources and subsequent education of rehabilitation staff, which, according to

Figure 3.2
Diagram of the transdisciplinary team from the TRU in Wigan (Jackson and Davies, 1995, with permission from Baillière Tindall)

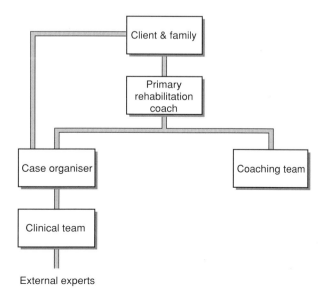

Jackson and Davies (1995), is prospectively cost-effective and increases levels of competency among the team as a whole. They also argue that the transdisciplinary model is most appropriate for rehabilitation of brain-injured clients, as it uses the clients' strengths to reduce handicap and increase quality of life.

Some central points to consider in the transdisciplinary approach are listed in Box 3.5.

Box 3.5
Central points of the interdisciplinary approach

- The clients' adaptive behaviours are focused upon.
- Flexibility of response is built in.
- Contact time with the client is greater.
- Errorless learning potential is increased.
- Clients may adversely become dependent on the primary therapist.
- Staff will need experience and training to cope with the responsibility as they move away from the more traditional methods of delivering care.
- A good understanding of all the team roles is essential.
- Caseload management is an essential feature.
- The role of the primary therapist should be clearly defined, in conjunction with the supportive team members' roles.

The diagrams in Figure 3.3 illustrate the main differences in the three team approaches.

Roles of team members

To have an effective rehabilitation team, it is important that each member of the team understands and respects each other's roles. The team members then have to build effective relationships between themselves in order for the team to work as a whole. The individual roles of team members will now be explored.

Figure 3.3
Diagrams of the communications links in the three different team approaches

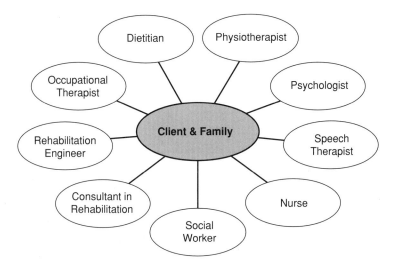

Figure 3.3a

Figure 3.3b

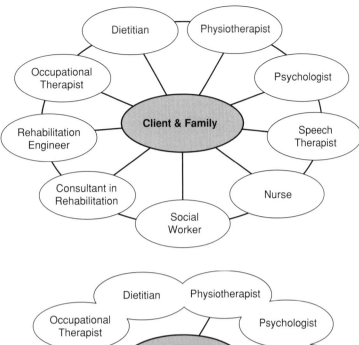

Figure 3.3c

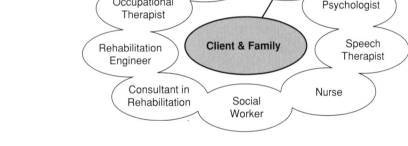

Medical staff   The doctor is an important member of the rehabilitation team and is often seen as the natural choice for team leader, both in terms of responsibility and expertise. The doctor is usually the first contact the client has before meeting the other team members. The doctor consults with and involves the rest of the team who work together to bring the client back to optimum health and independence. They assess clients' health status regularly. They explain diagnosis and prognosis to the client and relatives and often chair case conferences and other meetings. They are responsible for service development and audit and for fostering opportunities for staff education and the encouragement of research. They are increasingly involved in budgeting and management of the allocated resources alongside accountants and managers.

Nurses   Nurses constitute the biggest group within the health service and are a key aspect of the rehabilitation process (Chamberlain, 1988). Chamberlain recommends that it is the role of the ward manager/sister to influence the morale and ethos of the team of nurses on the unit. This may only be achieved by promoting an atmosphere of interdisciplinary teamwork, continuing communication, education and free expression of new ideas. It is important for the whole team to work together to achieve the set goals. Nurses also reinforce the other activities carried out by other members of the rehabilitation team and have a vital role to play in continuity of approach over the 24 hour-a-day, 7 day-a-week period. They achieve this by assessing clients' needs, planning care, delivering care, setting and reviewing goals in partnership with the client and relatives. Nurses maintain the clients' rights to privacy and dignity. They offer counselling and support to the client and to relatives. They are central to effective communication between all team members. They act as experts, especially in the areas of bowel and bladder management, skin care, wound care, pain management, nutrition and hydration and health promotion.

Rehabilitation nurses, in consultation with other team members, assist with assessment and management of many of the following areas:

- cognition
- positioning and wheelchair posture
- transfers
- medication
- sexuality
- teaching.

They work closely with other team members in discharge planning, along with the client and relatives.

Occupational therapist

Occupational therapy is defined as the treatment of physical and psychiatric conditions through specific activities, in order to help people reach a maximum level of function in all aspects of daily living (Curry and March, 1988). There are many aspects which the occupational therapists have to concentrate on and aim for in the area of client's daily living activities. The main aims of therapy are listed in Box 3.6.

Box 3.6
Main aims of occupational therapy

- To assess the difficulties a person has with the activities of daily living
- To facilitate maximum independence
- To encourage return to function and determine functional ability
- To help family and clients adjust to the new difficulties which will be encountered
- To prevent deformity
- To resettle the client in their home environment and in the real world, by arranging pre-discharge home visit or visits

- To provide the necessary aids and equipment to encourage independence
- To assess cognitive and perceptual problems

The occupational therapists work closely with the nursing staff and other disciplines within the unit environment to achieve the ultimate goals. They also liaise with the community services, rehabilitation engineer, and environmental control systems coordinator.

Physiotherapy

Physiotherapy is largely concerned with the improvement of function of the individual. The optimum results from physiotherapy are rarely achieved in isolation from other members of the team. The main aims of the physiotherapist are listed in Box 3.7.

Box 3.7
Main aims of the physiotherapist

- Strengthen muscle power
- Improve joint range, correct positioning, and functional movement training
- Improve neuromuscular coordination
- Improve cardiovascular efficiency and fitness
- Re-educate functional activity
- Use physical agents, such as ice and heat, to relieve secondary symptoms such as pain or muscle spasm

Education of client, relatives, carers and other team members is also an essential part of the physiotherapist's role.

Speech and language therapists

The role of speech therapists, as they are often referred to, varies according to their actual area of expertise. In general, they are mostly involved where clients have problems with dysphagia and communication. Early investigation of dysphagia is essential to prevent aspiration and aspirational pneumonia. Team members may refer directly to avoid delays. The speech therapist tests swallowing and advice is given to reduce risk of aspiration. They advise on positioning, consistency of the food and texture modification. They may advise further investigations (e.g. video fluoroscopy) if necessary, and in some areas, carry out this procedure themselves.

They assess aspects of communication and attempt to determine the type and extent of the problem, providing communication aids where appropriate. They also organise individual or group treatment and advise team members and relatives to reinforce and supplement information, and to practice exercises and approaches learnt in therapy sessions.

Speech therapists also play an important part in the education of ward staff and other professionals within the team, and in some areas, have established link workers to help ensure continued good practice.

Social workers   Social workers should become involved in the individual's care at an early stage when it becomes apparent that advice and support of social services will be required. It is vital to involve social services early, as arrangements can take a long time to make, and resources are notably hard to access. This includes setting up care and care packages, re-housing, adaptations and applying for grants and related disability benefits. The social service department is divided into areas usually with a disability team which helps with the following issues:

- practical assistance in the home with the help of the domiciliary care
- facilities at home, e.g. a hoist or commode
- recreational facilities for disabled people
- help with travelling facilities
- assistance in carrying out adaptation to the home
- assistance for holidays and respite care
- meals on wheels services
- extra equipment like a telephone and entry systems
- advice on application for benefits and grants.

Orthotist/ prosthetist   The Orthotist advises the team on the use of orthosis and other splints in clients with neurological disability, with the aim of improving function as a part of the rehabilitation of the individual. This may at times need to be a custom-made splint and require casting.

The prosthetist plays a major role in the rehabilitation of the amputee, and is involved with the early fitting of an initial prosthesis, and prescription of a definitive prosthesis, any modification to the prothesis, its fit and mechanical repairs and giving advice on change of prescription for appropriate function.

Clinical psychologist   Clinical psychologists are concerned with the assessment and management of cognitive problems in the client. They assist with assessment of anxiety and depression. They offer direct counselling to clients and relatives if required. They also offer this service to outpatients, as difficulties in adjustment and the extent of challenging behaviour are sometimes not apparent until after discharge. It is also acknowledged that other team members who are involved in managing clients with challenging behaviours will need guidance and support from the clinical psychologist.

Dietician   The dietician looks at the nutritional needs of the client and suggests special diets. The dietician also assesses the client by calculating the body mass index (BMI) and setting a target body weight. The dietician also liaises with the hospital kitchen staff to have special diets and meals prepared for clients. The dietician works closely with the nursing staff to advise and suggest suitable feeding regimes and nutritional intake: this will include issues around enteral feeding.

Rehabilitation engineer

The rehabilitation engineer assesses clients for special seating requirements, and in cases where problems have arisen with pressure relief. They are usually based at a wheelchair clinic or disability centre, and in most areas, they are able to attend the client in their own home if necessary. They usually work closely with the occupational therapists and physiotherapists.

Rehabilitation engineers are also employed on specialised projects, designing equipment for increasing independence and communication and environmental equipment advances.

Specialist nurses

Some units have specialist nurses attached to them. For example, at Hillingdon Hospital in London, the specialist nurse is a resource to the unit staff. They act as an expert or consultant, and ensure that current research reaches those working directly with the clients. They help the client and family to adjust to their new way of life and are usually involved in research and audit. Their primary role includes the evaluation and appraisal of current situations in order to obtain baseline data and the development of a programme such as an integrated care pathway (ICP), to assist in an interdisciplinary approach to rehabilitation. They also provide information, training and support for clients, carers and staff in the hospital and community settings.

Team building

If it is recognised that teamwork is vital in rehabilitation, then it is reasonable to expect that effort is required to build an effective team within the working environment. This will lead to improved efficiency and effectiveness in achieving the overall goals of the team member, the client and the organisation.

The responsibility for team building is not always explicit. It is arguably the domain of the ward sister or manager who has experience in this area, but it could be advanced by any senior team members, directors or in some instances, the clinical psychologist. Team building is a complex and major exercise, and time away from the workplace is often advocated (Dyer, 1994). Off-site events are often considered as unaffordable luxuries, but they do allow the advantage of less interruption from clients, phone calls and other colleagues.

Topics for team discussion should be chosen by the group; an internal or external facilitator would assist the process. There is a tendency to over-complicate the team building process (Eales-White,

1996). One way to avoid this could be to keep the group sessions informal, comfortable and group-led. Brainstorming is a useful method of sharing ideas, it also promotes communication, breaks down hierarchical barriers and allows a problem-solving approach to be utilised. It is vital for team members to become mutually support-ive and trusting of each other's abilities, in order to develop as an effective team. This includes resolving interpersonal attitudes, agree-ing on the team objectives, and the development of the task mission or vision. Therefore, if the teams' mission is to successfully reinteg-rate the individual client into the community setting, while achieving optimum independence, this should be linked to the team building strategy. The success of team building is also dependent on regular review, feedback and support mechanisms, which may be agreed locally, and will assist the team to assess its own effectiveness.

Team building is a continuous process. It should focus on setting goals, communication, decision-making and interpersonal relation-ships. The success of team building interventions should also be measurable, which means that certain problems are overcome, for example:

- confusion as to roles and relationships within the team is lessened
- members clearly understand short-term functional goals
- the team mission is agreed upon
- personal development is encouraged.

Wood (1993), in his work on the rehabilitation team, points out that effective functioning of the team will include achievement of oper-ational goals as well as personal development, which are seen as inseparable in teamwork. This requires further attention, as it is seen to affect overall team performance. Team performance has been researched extensively, and the literature available should be utilised as a valuable background to those studying team dynamics and development.

Performance appraisal

Conducting performance appraisals is a convenient way of identify-ing individual team members' needs and reviewing these in terms of the demands made by the organisation. Kakabadse, Ludlow and Vinnicombe (1988) looked at the work of Dr Shaun Tyson and Alfred York, and concluded that there are five reasons for carrying out performance appraisals:

- to determine people's suitability and potential for particular types of employment
- to look at the individual's training and development needs
- to address aspirations and promotional prospects
- to give time and feedback on performance aiming to develop motivation and commitment
- to discuss reward.

Performance appraisal is seen as a two-way process: the individual has the opportunity to discuss aims and achievements, skills, and problems encountered; the appraiser looks at the appraisees contribution to the team. Taking a participative approach, whereby they meet informally and exchange ideas and views on each other's performance is recommended (Kakabadse et al., 1988). They also suggest basic requirements, again from the work of Tyson and York, which should be encompassed in the appraisal approach. These include:

- work performance, experience, educational needs and aims and objectives
- uniform use throughout the organisation
- understanding by all employees
- training for managers in application of the system.

There are some examples of good practice in certain areas, where appraisals are conducted effectively and sensitively, which show that they are an effective method of assessing performance and linking this to individual and organisational objectives. The experience of the district rehabilitation unit at The Hillingdon Hospital, London, which has a rotational post of senior registrar in conjunction with the regional rehabilitation unit at Northwick Park Hospital, is one such example. In these units, the senior registrar is appraised by the consultants of both units and the unit manager. This idea was developed by Dr Lynne Turner-Stokes, Director of the Regional Rehabilitation Unit, Northwick Park Hospital, London. Interest has been expressed in adopting the idea nationwide. A similar appraisal system is also considered relevant to other specialities with a multidisciplinary approach, for example, palliative medicine. This system has been brought about by the need for the physician to be recognised as a member of the team. The need for medical skills to be reviewed alongside teamworking is seen as an essential part of the registrars' training. Objectives and goals should be set to ensure continuity throughout the placement.

Performance review is one method of motivating the individual to achieve personal and organisational goals, and it is an integral part of team building. Managers should develop the idea of interdisciplinary appraisal, as they can thus help to foster the development of teamwork in this important area.

Communication

Communication is the sharing of necessary information between people concerned with achievements of the team's objectives. In the rehabilitation setting, this can be between clients, team members, relatives and other professionals, or any combination of the above. Bakheit (1996) states that the main objectives of communication are:

- to convey information
- to receive feedback, in order to effect change.

Bakheit also recommends ways to improve communication: keep the message brief and clear, avoid ambiguity, avoid the use of professional jargon, and use both formal and informal channels of communication.

There are several keys to improving interdisciplinary communication worth mentioning. Meetings, for instance, are needed to facilitate formal communication. Team members do need to spend regular time together, although this is often not seen as a priority, due to heavy workloads and shortage of time and staff. For the team to coordinate effort effectively, it must spend time communicating, therefore attendance at team meetings should be insisted upon.

Ideally, staff working in teams should be located in close proximity to each other. This should be borne in mind especially where staff are members of other departments, for example, speech therapists or social workers. They are often housed away from the rehabilitation unit in a departmental office. This can make team building difficult and ideally is to be avoided where possible.

Developments in the use of interdisciplinary documentation are seen as a method of fostering good communication. Many areas are developing their own case note systems. These are usually created in-house by the team members themselves. All team members are able to contribute to the record of clients' care. They include documentation of treatment, nursing care, any investigations, therapy problems, goals, and future plans.

Integrated documentation has several advantages which can possibly simplify and improve health care generally. They are time saving, although it is recognised that separate disciplines persist in keeping their own records of care, possibly for their own security, which is not always seen as serving the client's interest. It certainly makes sense for separate contributions to care from each discipline when they are recorded in one set of documentation. This allows for logical progression which is timely and based on interdisciplinary goals. Conscientious recording and commitment to integrated documentation is essential if all team members are to benefit from this approach. Client benefit can also be shown, as any member of the team has up-to-date information regarding investigations, therapy management and progress. This is particularly useful to nurses working on shifts who have little contact with the therapists in question.

There is growing interest in developing interdisciplinary documentation, and many places are implementing or piloting such innovative practice, for example, the 'Mudipors', developed and used at the Regional Rehabilitation Unit, Northwick Park Hospital, London and

'Acorns' (Alderbourne Combined Rehabilitation Notes) developed and used at Hillingdon Hospital Rehabilitation Unit, London.

Integrated care pathways

Integrated care pathways (ICPs) are best described as a tool for improving the quality of care delivered. They are a form of case management which is becoming increasingly popular in this country, following their introduction in the early 1990s from the USA.

ICPs involve the whole rehabilitation team, both in their formation, which should be led by the local professionals who deliver the care, and in their implementation and subsequent analysis. An ICP assists the team members in the coordination of care by identifying the activities which must occur to reach the standards or quality of care which has been predetermined. These activities are set out in a consecutive and synchronised fashion to achieve a coordinated interdisciplinary approach. The ICP document may be held by the client. It is informative and can give the client, or relative where appropriate, an idea of what to expect. It is hoped that this in turn allows the client to gain more control of their position and encourages empowerment, contribution and cooperation.

One criticism of ICPs is that patients may find the documents difficult to read. Another disadvantage frequently encountered is the perception that ICPs involve additional paperwork. In practice, though, the opposite may be found. If this is not found to be the case, then it may well be a fault within the care path itself, and can be reviewed and changed, if necessary, to reflect the needs of the client group concerned. Setting up an ICP is time-consuming, however, the time invested is a worthwhile learning and staff training process. Interdisciplinary differences can be resolved at this early stage. Furthermore, when it comes to writing another ICP, it is easier the second and third time around.

In the current climate of health care, we are constantly being asked to account for what we do and how we do it. The ICP is a tool, which involves the whole rehabilitation team, for clinical audit. Variance analysis is an in-built audit tool. A variance is defined as a detour from patient care activities as outlined in the ICP. A variance is not a failure, although this did appear to be a source of concern to many professionals, especially when first introduced. The services of a good facilitator can be of immeasurable assistance in this case. The variance analysis provides us with the audit data, information which can then be used to influence practice development, review performance, and provide local solutions to identified areas of concern.

ICPs and variance analysis need not be difficult to achieve. They can promote teamwork and improve interdisciplinary communication, as well as cross professional boundaries. Finally, ICPs are infinitely shareable between settings, and can foster links nationally as we all strive to improve the quality of care delivered to our client

Figure 3.4a

An integrated care pathway for planned short stay/assessment used in the Hillingdon Hospital District Rehabilitation Unit for clients with neurological illness

Admit. date:.........................

Disch. date:.........................

Diagnosis:.........................

Admitting Nurse:.........................

Date	Day	Variance	Source	Action taken	Comments	Initials

Code 1–14

(+) positive variance
(–) negative variance

Coding guidelines:

1 Patient unwell
2 Patient not available
3 Awaiting assessment
4 Other assessment

= anticipated variance faster than expected
= anticipated variance slower than expected
5 Awaiting outcome
6 Investigation results awaited
7 Arranged
8 Not arranged

9 Satisfactory
10 Unsatisfactory
11 Patient refused
12 Clinically not indicated

13 Staff not available
14 Appropriate staff not available

Figure 3.4b

Keyworker: ....

Team: ....

Day	Medical	Nursing	Therapies	Others
1 **Mon**	1 Initial clerking 2 Arrange nec. investigations 3 Assess prescription/medication 4 ± refer to other specialities 5 Confirm list of MDT goals (please list below)	1 Orientation to ward by Keyworker/admitting nurse 2 Check pre-admission sheet from relatives/carers 3 Check if DV/OP, etc. Report 4 Give information leaflet to patient 5 Give psychological support 6 Baseline obs. – bowels, temp., BP, respiration 7 Waterlow scoring 8 Liaise with OT 9 Liaise with PT 10 ± refer to Psychologist 11 ± refer to Speech Therapist 12 Inform doctor of patient's arrival 13 Routine nursing care	1 Introduction to PT 2 Introduction to OT	1 Medical Records available 2 ACoRn insert – Ward Clerk 3 ICP insert – Ward Clerk

Routine nursing care: 1) Bathing 2) Toileting 3) Medication 4) Assist with nutritional needs 5) Skin care

Figure 3.4c

| 2 | | 1 Start FIM/FAM
2 Check body weight
3 Nutritional Assessment
4 Refer to Dietitian
5 Urine analysis
6 Routine nursing care | | 1 Assessment by PT
– PT assessment
– PT problem list
– Formulate PT treatment regime
– FIM/FAM

2 Initial interview by OT
– OT problem list from patient/carer
– Formulate OT treatment programme
– Identify wh. ch. problem
– + inform Rehab. Engineer (wh. ch. problem)

3 Speech Therapy assessment
– Dysphagia
– Speech/language
– SpT problem list
– SpT report and advice
– SpT ± FIM/FAM | Dietitian assessment |
| 3 | 1 ± routine medical review
2 ± check investigation results | 1 + refer to SW
2 + refer to Chiropody
3 FIM/FAM
4 Routine nursing care | | 1 PT session
2 OT – start assessment
3 OT – ECE assessment
4 OT – check home situation
5 OT – liaison with community team
6 OT – FIM/FAM score | |

Routine nursing care: 1) Bathing 2) Toileting 3) Medication 4) Assist with nutritional needs (5) Skin care

Figure 3.4d

			Ward round	Clinical Psychology assessment
4	Ward round 1 Check results of investigations 2 Record in medical notes 3 Complete FIM/FAM 4 Confirm combined problem list 5 Identify multidisp. goals (please list below)	Ward round 1 Routine nursing care	1 PT session 2 PT liaison with carer 3 OT ± arrange Home Visit 4 OT continue treatment sessions 5 OT liaison with carer 6 FIM/FAM discussion	± Chiropody
5	Routine medical review	Routine nursing assessment	1 PT session 2 OT session 3 SpT session	
6		Routine nursing care		
7		Routine nursing care		
8	Routine medical review	Weekend report to doctor Routine nursing care	1 PT session/evaluation and treatment 2 OT session	± Clinical Psychology session
9		Routine nursing care	1 PT session 2 OT session 3 SpT session 4 SpT summary for Discharge letter	

Routine nursing care: 1) Bathing   2) Toileting   3) Medication   4) Assist with nutritional needs   5) Skin care

Figure 3.4e

	Medical	Nursing	Therapy	Discharge/Admin
10	Routine medical review	Routine nursing care	1 PT session/discharge plan 2 OT session/finalising assessment	
11	**Ward round** 1 Final FIM/FAM score for 2 Discharge plan 3 Discuss next admission date 4 TTA 5 Other follow-up appointments 6 Medical review 7 Arrange next admission	**Ward round** 1 Arrange TTA 2 Book transport 3 Liaise with carer 4 Liaise with DN 5 Liaise with SW 6 Arrange next admission 7 ± liaison with relative/carers	**Ward round** FIM/FAM revision	**Ward round** ± Clinical Psychology summary for Discharge letter
12		Routine nursing care Liaison with relative/carers	1 PT session 2 OT session 3 SpT session	
13		Routine nursing care		
14		Routine nursing care		
15	Discharge GP letter	Routine nursing care Complete discharge check list	Discharge	Discharge – Ward Manager to check Medical Records in preparation for Disch. Summary → Doctor Next admission – Ward Clerk/Secretary onto PSS waiting list/index card

Routine nursing care: 1) Bathing 2) Toileting 3) Medication 4) Assist with nutritional needs 5) Skin care

group. Figure 3.4 is a sample of one ICP currently in use for planned short stay assessment of patients with neurological illness in a rehabilitation unit.

Goal setting

Although goal setting is explored in detail in Chapter 6, it is relevant to discuss it to a degree in this chapter in relation to team-working.

Much consideration has been given to the role of goals in directing, and even manipulating human behaviour (Gross, 1990; Hargie and Marshall, 1989; Vroom and Deci, 1992), whether in the form of needs (Maslow, 1972), drives (Hull, 1943), or in order to relieve tensions (Lewin, 1951). Probably the most influential theorist in the field is Locke (1976), who postulated an entire theory proposing that an individual's conscious goals are the primary determinants of behaviour. Goal setting is simply the process of establishing these goals. However, the term is most often used to indicate a process not only of determining goals, but also of optimising conditions for their definition, planning for their achievement and the systematic steps involved in their execution.

The purpose of goal setting generally, is to act as a motivator to increase performance or reach targets, however, it can have many additional benefits. For example, when used in the team setting it can serve to coordinate its members. Its application can help to:

■ increase job performance
■ assist in personal development
■ set organisational goals
■ set personal goals
■ set goals for the client in the health care setting.

Locke describes the attributes of the mental processes involved in goal setting as being: goal specificity (degree of quantitative precision of the goal), goal difficulty (level of performance sought), goal intensity (process of setting goal and means to reach it), and goal commitment (amount of effort required to achieve goal), (Gibson, Ivanievich and Donnely, 1994).

Goal setting can be used by the skilled manager to enhance the performance of the work force. Latham and Locke (1979) suggest that goal setting as a means of directing a workforce towards organisational objectives is probably not only more effective than other methods but may be a major mechanism by which other incentives effect motivation. However, although they state in their paper that goal setting alone increases performance, they themselves found in their studies that goal setting had to be coupled with supervisory presence. Verbal praise was also a further variant. This, perhaps should be borne in mind.

Goal setting, especially from a managerial perspective, should include the stages outlined in Box 3.8. It is suggested that ignoring any of the stages will lead to failure (Gibson et al., 1994).

Box 3.8
The main stages in goal setting

- Diagnoses, i.e. whether the people, organisation and technology are suited to goal planning
- Preparing, or readying employees
- Emphasizing, and ensuring that key aspects of goal setting are understood by managers and subordinates
- Conducting a review of the situation in order that necessary alterations can be made to reach goals
- Performing a final review to check goals set, are modified and accomplished

As the interdisciplinary team is central to rehabilitation, so goal planning is pivotal to the effectiveness of the interdisciplinary team. Reduction of handicap in clients with complex needs requires input from a variety of disciplines. These disciplines need to work together as an integrated whole. When goal planning is not interdisciplinary, individual disciplines may aim for goals which duplicate one another, conflict with each other or do not improve the overall general life functioning of the client (McGrath and Davis, 1992). In this context, goal setting is a process of creative problem-solving. The procedure may vary according to the team involved, and many models have been suggested to isolate the key stages involved. These include five stages put forward by McGrath and Davis (1992), a 'machine model' of human problem solving (Newell and Simon, 1963) and a comprehensive model proposed by Powell et al. (1994). However, interdisciplinary client-centered goal setting in the rehabilitation environment can generally be thought of as having the same overall key components:

- recognition of the overall goal or philosophy of the rehabilitation team
- identification of the long-term aims of treatment
- classification and analysis of short-term goals
- task appropriation and reduction
- activation and evaluation.

Short-term goals must be allocated to the most suitable discipline, which undoubtedly must involve collaboration between disciplines.

The team must, however, decide on means of goal attainment, as working towards the same goal using different approaches could be very confusing to the client. This is where the role of a designated key-worker can be used to complement the team approach. The key-worker may be from any discipline involved in the client's care.

They are usually the team member who has the most input into planning that care, but this method of allocation may vary from area to area. It is important that the key-worker understands their role within the team, and also that they are able to explain this to the client and relatives. Essential aspects of the key-worker's role are listed in Box 3.9.

Box 3.9
Essential duties of the key-worker in rehabilitation

- Be the primary communicator with client, family and carers
- Discuss the rehabilitation process with the above
- Allow time for discussion of any fears or concerns they may have
- Liaise, and feedback information to all team members, relatives and the client
- Liaise with relevant outside agencies
- Keep the team informed of developments/changes in the rehabilitation programme or condition of the patient
- Ensure all information is documented
- Keep oneself informed and updated
- Review current situation as appropriate
- Initiate assessments and referrals
- Initiate treatment plan/goals, involving client and interdisciplinary team
- Complete documentation that is not discipline-specific
- Arrange all meetings (i.e. case conferences, professional and social meetings and appointments)
- Plan means of achievement of goals (i.e. who does what, how and when)

Finally, regular meetings are required to assess goal attainment and to restructure goals where required. Successful meetings should achieve the desired results; decisions may need to be made, all team members have the opportunity to contribute. It is hoped that in this way, a balanced view and hoped-for result is reached.

Conclusion

This chapter has focused on the effective rehabilitation team. It has attempted to give an overview of the different models of team organisation, in order that the practitioner may consider these and adapt and apply them to their own setting as appropriate. Roles of team members are described, and can be used to gain further understanding of each other's roles, however, this does not replace experience in the field. Developments such as integrated care pathways and integrated case notes must take place concurrently with increasing awareness of the importance of team-building, establishment of a clear vision, and application of goal setting processes to enhance the effective team approach in the rehabilitation setting.

Successful teamwork is not easy to achieve. It is important to acknowledge theories of teamwork, and apply these principles to practice, to assist team development and to improve performance. An action plan will help team development and in the implementation of change. An action plan may also produce evidence of effective teamwork. Individual areas may develop personalised action plans based on their own ideas and systems of beliefs. The desired outcome of the action plan overall should include improved delivery of service to clients, which is measurable, and that team members will feel supported in their work, developed, highly motivated, satisfied and possessing a team spirit, to achieve increased cooperation and trust between themselves. Some suggestions of items to include in a comprehensive action plan for successful teamworking are listed in Box 3.10.

Box 3.10
Suggested items for planning teamworking

- Agree objectives – Aim for quality of care, use of resources and operational policies
- Understand each other's roles
- Interdisciplinary education – include education on teamwork issues
- Develop people – within the organisation, the team and its leaders
- Ensure effective communication
- Develop the key-worker role
- Evaluate – measurement and audit
- Team briefings and meetings
- Enjoyment and reward – professional trust and friendship are essential

It may seem that the rehabilitation team has a great deal of ground to cover in order to achieve effective delivery of care to clients. It is true to say that successful teamwork can be considered as a measurable contribution and a rewarding experience for all involved.

Questions for discussion

- What are the key components of an effective team?
- Is it possible to define which features of teamwork are responsible for improved patient outcome?
- Can tools such as integrated care pathways be considered useful in promoting interdisciplinary teamwork?

Acknowledgement

I would like to thank all my team, especially Melanie Williams, Jane Hubble, Dr Rajiv Hanspal, Sue Barron, Aleks de Gromoboy, Anne Costelloe and David Whitelock for their contributions and help with this chapter.

References

Bakheit, A. (1996) Effective teamwork in rehabilitation. *International Journal of Rehabilitation Research*, **19**, 301–306.

Blake, R. & Mouton, J. (1964) *The Management Grid*. Houston, Texas: The Gulf Publication Company.

Brill, N. I. (1976) *Teamwork: Working Together in the Human Services*. Philadelphia: JB Lippincott.

Chamberlain, M.A. (1988) The rehabilitation team and functional assessment. In *Rehabilitation of the Physically Disabled Adult*, eds. Goodwill, C.I. & Chamberlain, M.A. London: Croom Helm.

Curry, R. & March, H. (1988) Occupational therapy. In *Rehabilitation of the Physically Disabled Adult*, eds. Goodwill, C.J. & Chamberlain M.A. London: Croom Helm.

Dingwall, R. (1980) Problems of teamwork in primary care. In *Teamwork in the Personal Social Services and Health Care*. London: Croom Helm.

Dyer, W.G. (1984) *Team Building: Issues and Alternatives*. Reading MA: Addison-Wesley.

Eales-White, R. (1996) *Building your Team*. London: Kogan Page Limited.

Embling, S. (1995) Exploring multidisciplinary teamwork. *British Journal of Therapy and Rehabilitation*, **2**, 142–144.

Furnell, J., Flett, S. & Clarke, D.F. (1987) Multidisciplinary clinical teams: some issues in establishment and function. *Hospital and Health Services Review*, 15–18.

Gibson, J.L., Ivanievich, J.M. & Donnely, E.H.Jnr. (1994) *Organisations: Behaviour, Structure, Process*, 8th edn. USA: R. D. Irwin.

Gross, R.D. (1990) *Psychology: the Science of Mind and Behaviour*. London: Hodder and Stoughton.

Hargie, O. & Marshall, P. (1989) Interpersonal Communication: a Theoretical Framework. In *A Handbook of Communication Skills*, ed. Hargie, O. London: Routledge.

Hull, C.L. (1943) *Principles of Behaviour*. New York: Appleton-Century-Crofts.

Jackson, H. & Davies, M. (1995) A transdisciplinary approach to brain injury rehabilitation. *British Journal of Therapy and Rehabilitation*, **2**, 65–70.

Kakabadse, A., Ludlow, R. & Vinnicombe, S. (1988) *Working in Organisations*. London: Penguin Books.

Latham, G.P. & Locke, G.A. (1979) Goal-setting: a motivational technique that works. In *Management and Motivation*, eds. Vroom, V.H. & Deci, E.L. Middlesex: Penguin.

Leland, M., Lewis, F.D., Hinman, S., Carrillo, R. (1988) Functional retraining of traumatically brain-injured adults in a transdisciplinary environment. *Rehabilitation Counselling* **31**, 289–297.

Lewin, K. (1951) Intension, will and need. In *Organisation and Pathology of Thought*, ed. Rapaport, D. pp. 95–153. New York: Columbia University Press.

Locke, E.A. (1976) The nature and causes of job satisfaction. In *Handbook of Industrial and Organisational Psychology*, ed. Dunnette, M.D. pp. 1297–1394. USA: Rand McNally.

McGrath, J. & Davis, A. (1992) Rehabilitation: where we are going and how do we get there? *Clinical Rehabilitation*, **6**, 225–235.

Mandy, P. (1996) Interdisciplinary rather than multidisciplinary or generic practice. *British Journal of Therapy and Rehabilitation*, **3**, 110–112.

Maslow, A. (1972) *The Farther Reaches of Human Nature*. New York: The Viking Press.

Muir-Giles, G. & Clark-Wilson, J. (1993) *Brain Injury Rehabilitation: A Neurofunctional Approach*. London: Chapman and Hall.

Newell, A. & Simon, H.A. (1963) *G.P.S. a Programme that Stimulates Human Thought*, pp. 279–293. New York: McGraw Hill.

Ovretveit, J. (1986) *Organisation of Multidisciplinary Clinical Teams*. Uxbridge: Brunel University Health Services Centre.

Petrie, H.G. (1976) Do you see what I see? The epistemology of interdisciplinary inquiry. *Journal of Anaesthetic Education* **10**, 29–43.

Pfeiffer, S.I. (1980) The school-based interprofessional team: recurring problems and some possible solutions. *Journal of School Psychology*, **18**, 388–394.

Powell, T. et al. (1994) An interdisciplinary approach to the rehabilitation of people with brain injury. *British Journal of Therapy and Rehabilitation*, **1**, 8–13.

Sachs, P.R. (1991) *Treating Families of Brain-Injured Survivors.* New York: Springer.

Vroom, V.H. & Deci, E.L. eds. (1992) *Management and Motivation.* Middlesex: Penguin.

Wood, R. (1993) The rehabilitation team. In *Neurological Rehabilitation,* eds. Greenwood R. et al., Ch. 4. Edinburgh: Churchill Livingstone.

Further reading

Adair, J. (1987) *Effective Team Building.* London: Pan Books.

Easy to read, with useful lists of desirable attributes of team members and considerations for a well functioning team.

Belbin, M.R. (1981) *Management Teams: Why they Succeed or Fail.* London: Heinemann.

Essential reading, with good descriptions and definitions.

Brill, N.I. (1976) *Teamwork.* New York: J.B. Lippincott Co.

Good definitions.

Dawson, J. & Barlett, E. (1996) Change within interdisciplinary teamwork: one unit's experience. *British Journal of Therapy and Rehabilitation,* 6, 225–235.

Fielder, F.E. & Chemers, M.M. (1974) *Leadership and Effective Management.* New York: Scott Foresman and Company.

Marguerison, C. & McCann, R. (1990) *Team Management: Practical New Approaches.* London: WH Allen & Co.

See Chapters 7 and 9 on action plans and high performing teams.

Rosen, N. (1989) *Teamwork and the Bottom Line: Groups Make a Difference.* Hillsdale, New Jersey: Lawrence Erlbaum Associates.

Look at the Task Group Effectiveness Inventory, and chapter on The Manager.

CARE PLANNING AND REHABILITATION

4 Assessment in rehabilitation

Iain Bowie

Key issues
- Scope of assessment
- Assessment methods
- Specific assessment measures
- Problem-related assessment

Introduction

This chapter introduces the concept and practice of client assessment in rehabilitation. A brief examination of the nature of assessment within rehabilitation is followed by a section on the scope and practice of nursing assessment. The third major section concerns some of the specific assessment practices that may be performed in rehabilitation. There are some illustrative case studies adapted from real client histories and a short section to recommend further reading.

Assessment is usually recognised as the first stage of the problem-solving approach. Whatever model of care is practised, assessment will probably be the first activity of the health care professionals. Assessment (or some aspect of it) comes first in very different types of care settings, whether this is in the form of triage of wounded soldiers in battle, or diagnostic examination by a physician, or assessment of a client referred for a mobility aid. Interventions need to be based on the outcome of results of an assessment.

In rehabilitation practice, there are some additional points to consider which emphasise the importance of accurate and effective assessment. These include cognitive or communication deficits where the routine assessment of the client is complicated by their 'impaired' contribution. Rehabilitation is usually defined in terms of facilitating the restoration of optimum function in the biopsychosocial aspects of the client's life. Clients who require physical rehabilitation will have specific needs in biological terms, activities of everyday living, psychological needs and social needs. For clients with severe physical and cognitive disabilities following disease or trauma, assessment will have to ensure that these needs are addressed in the subsequent rehabilitative care. Where communication is impaired, assessment has to be based on a reduced battery of techniques, so eliciting information requires a highly skilled level of practice.

Nursing is not the only discipline involved in rehabilitation, and consequently, nurses are involved in assessment in two layers of interaction. First, nurses assess the specific nursing requirements of the client, such as (using terms from the Roper model) maintaining body temperature and so on. In this role, the nurse must assess the client and devise the plan of nursing care. Nurses are also responsible for contributing their unique skills and knowledge as part of the interdisciplinary team. Additionally, nurses are present around the clock in practice settings. Nurses are often the first members of the team that meet a new client. They are in a unique position to liaise with various team members and the family and friends of the client. In this role, the nurse must assess the client in terms of nursing needs, as one of the aspects of the rehabilitation process. Speech and language therapists, occupational therapists and physiotherapists are among other key professionals who may contribute to the process.

Figure 4.1 shows how aspects of nursing assessment interlock with the other disciplines to produce a team rehabilitation plan. It is, of course, entirely diagrammatic and there are many other aspects of nursing and the therapies which would need to be included in a comprehensive assessment. Each of the therapies will make their own professional assessment and it may include different techniques for dealing with different aspects of the disability. In turn, the nurse

Figure 4.1
Nursing as part of the multidisciplinary team

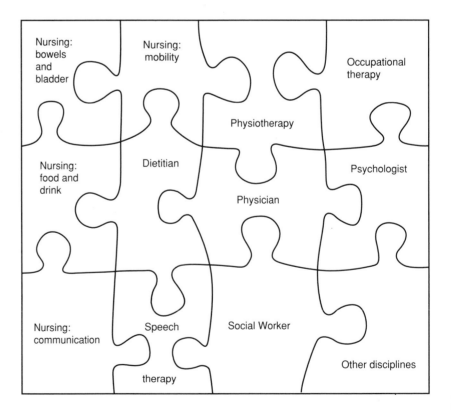

Figure 4.2
Nursing assessment summary

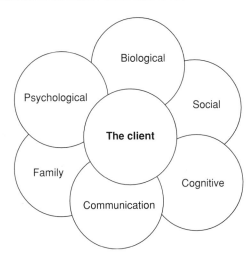

may assess in areas relevant to nursing expertise, such as those exemplified in the diagram. There are many other areas of nursing, such as skin care or self medication, that have been omitted for simplicity, so the real jigsaw might have many more pieces.

Nursing assessment traditionally involves several separate systems which are summarised in Figure 4.2. There are other models and methods of representing this, but Figure 4.2 shows the main areas of concern to nursing professionals. Individual items within each of the overlapping circles will be further developed later in this chapter. In the future, the use of integrated care pathways may simplify multiple assessments by use of collaborative care programs. These will amalgamate all the anticipated elements of care and treatment from all members of the multidisciplinary team.

Nursing assessment is based on standard models of practice and varies with the location of care. Most nurses are familiar with care models and practice according to established systems.

Standard models of practice used in rehabilitation nursing include Roper's activities of living model, which is well known in the UK and forms the basis of the textbook edited by Hoeman (1996). Orem's self-care model is also widely practised in rehabilitation units, because of the basis of the development of self-care for the client (Knust and Quarn, 1983). A third model used in rehabilitation is Roy's adaptation model (Gless, 1995; Piazza and Foote, 1990), where adaptation to health and ill health is emphasised. The Peplau model, which emphasises the development of the therapeutic relationship between the nurse and client, has also been used in a rehabilitation context (Jones, 1995).

Many units build their own models and some integrate features of standard models to suit their own specific requirements. It is within the framework of these models that the assessment of the client has to take place. Therefore, it is important to establish an assessment system that reflects the model that is practised, and vice versa.

Assessment itself, as an aspect of rehabilitation, may include features that are fairly general in scope, such as functional assessment routines, or it may be very specific and just look at one aspect of the client's requirements. Examples of this latter kind are scales such as the Ashworth spasticity scale or HAD (Hospital Anxiety and Depression). By using a battery of these assessment techniques, the rehabilitation team can build up a picture of the client. Not all assessment tests are necessary for all clients to provide a comprehensive picture from which to plan the rehabilitation program. It is necessary to select those assessment measures that will provide the information required for the care of each individual client.

Box 4.1
Reasons for assessment

- It forms the basis of the rehabilitation program and nursing care planning.
- It forms a baseline against which progress can be monitored.
- It indicates the level of severity of the problem.
- Nursing diagnosis is related to assessment findings (see chapter 5).
- It provides useful follow-up data after discharge.
- It provides a set of data for research purposes.
- It can be used to select clients who are suitable for rehabilitation and the type of rehabilitation that is best for them (pre-admission assessment).
- It can provide data for suitability and provision of assistive devices (eating aids, wheelchairs and so on).
- It can be used to select a suitable compensatory technique or skill to be taught to clients and family.
- It is performed as part of a transfer procedure to another placement or discharge to the community.
- Assessment can be used to estimate the dependency of the patient and hence workload.
- Quality assurance programs and audit can be measured against gathered assessment data.
- It can be used as a tool in skill mix studies.

For the reasons listed in Box 4.1, assessment forms the foundation of all care and can affect the care of other clients in the future. As evidence-based practice in health care becomes established in modern practice, the information from client assessment and progress forms the backbone of research and future practice.

Scope of assessment

The source of the data (see Box 4.2) is important and as mentioned earlier, may be problematic for rehabilitation nurses.

Box 4.2
Typical sources of data

- ■ the client
- ■ friends and family
- ■ medical records and transfer documents
- ■ diagnostic tests such as blood chemistry, haematology, micro-biology, imaging and physiological function tests (electro-encephalogram, or spirometry)
- ■ functional and physical test batteries and assessment scales

Assessment by nurses usually follows the pattern dictated by the model of practice in local use. All nursing models will probably cover similar aspects of the client's care in one way or another. It is up to the nursing team to establish the most suitable for use in their own unit. These aspects of care are listed and discussed below.

Cognitive

The client's cognitive abilities are of great importance when assessing: not only to choose the appropriate intervention, but also to establish the reliability of the information that the client supplies. The client's memory and attention span may interfere with accurate data collection. Dysphasia (discussed below) will limit the amount the client can contribute in giving a history, however, the patient may well have normal speech and still have memory loss or exhibit dementia.

Communication

It is a priority to assess communication early in the process, so that the remainder of the assessment can be completed. If the client is dysphasic, the assessment procedure will have to take this into account. Cognitive and communication deficits may overlap in conditions such as locked-in syndrome. In the first instance, it may delay care to wait for the professional assessment of the speech and language therapists. With this in mind, the nurse may assess the client's verbal expression and understanding. There are a number of simple standard tests where the communicative ability is assessed (described later in this chapter). The nurse should be able to distinguish between dysphasia (expressive, receptive or global), dyspraxia and dysarthria because the effectiveness of nurse–client communication depends on identifying the language or speech deficits. Deaf people with dysphasia will have impaired signing ability. Other cognitive problems, such as poor memory or neglect, may produce results similar to dysphasia. Deafness and visual impairment may also present problems when assessing the client because they may interfere with the outcome criteria of a test. Motor impairment may result in dysarthria.

Mobility and movement

Like communication, mobility and movement are essential for other aspects of daily life. Therefore, an early assessment of these key areas will provide information about the client's ability to perform other activities. Patterns of paralysis or weakness should be noted. Tremor, rigidity, spasticity and contractures also interfere with mobility and normal movement, and should be assessed. More detailed professional assessment by the physiotherapists is fundamental in many instances and much of the information needed for the care plan can be obtained by the physiotherapists.

Activities of daily living

Many of the activities of daily living are professionally assessed by the occupational therapy team. Nurses need to assess the client's ability to wash, groom, dress, feed and go to the toilet. Apart from the rehabilitative (that is, maximising function) element of care, nurses need to establish the amount of nursing support necessary.

Social factors

Social factors in care are usually more difficult to assess due to their intangible nature (see Box 4.3). Social factors may also take longer to assess because of this intangible nature and reliance on difficult communication. It may be tempting to leave social assessment till last, or to omit it. However, if assessment is taken as the first step in providing a comprehensive rehabilitation program, it is essential that these issues are addressed early on in the assessment phase.

Box 4.3
Social items that have to be assessed

- client's family
- socialisation
- finance
- vocational prospects
- educational background and needs
- home circumstances
- sexual circumstances
- religious and spiritual beliefs

Psychological

The psychological status is also very important, because it provides a framework for care. Psychological assessment will include the perception of illness, coping strategies, anxiety, depression, and behavioural problems such as eating disorders, aggression and disinhibition. The nurse will need to observe the client's sleep patterns and behaviour. Sensory and motor impairment can affect psychological status causing mood swings and depression. Drugs used in treatment may cause psychological 'side-effects', such as steroid psychosis.

Assessment methods

Assessment can be both subjective or objective. A subjective observation relies on the observation of the client or professional of, for example, physical appearance or reported pain. An objective observation is independent of individual 'opinion' and relies on instruments or 'paper tools'. Assessment scales are an example of 'paper tools'. They have been developed to aid assessment and produce reliable, valid, sensitive and easily applicable techniques. Most nurses are familiar with the concept of scales for assessing risk or functional level. The Norton, Braden and Waterlow scales are widely used for predicting the risk of pressure ulcers. The Glasgow coma scale is used internationally to estimate level of consciousness. In rehabilitation practice, there are several scales in use. Other techniques include physical examination, vital signs, electrical and chemical tests and body imaging. Any objective technique must fulfil several criteria before it is accepted (see Box 4.4).

Box 4.4
Criteria for objective assessment techniques

Reliability	It should give consistent, reproducible results. A good example of a reliable test is use of a thermometer. Provided it is used correctly, it will give the same result regardless of who performs the test. Inter-rater reliability is the consistency of results obtained by two or more assessors.
Validity	The test should measure what it is supposed to measure. The radial pulse rate is a valid measure of heart rate as it accurately reflects heart rate (though not entirely reliable in heart failure, when radial and apex beat is sometimes performed).
Sensitivity	The measure should pick up changes. One criticism of some of the pressure ulcer risk scales is that they over-predict, that is, more people are placed in the 'at risk' category than is reflected by the incidence of pressure ulcers.
Sensibility	This refers to the appropriateness of the test for the 'function' to be assessed.

(Lumley and Benjamin, 1994)

An excellent table concerning the reliability and validity of assessment instruments is found in Gresham et al. (1995). This table is fully referenced (see Further Reading).

Details of these criteria are available in journals and text books that describe the assessment methods. Before selecting a particular assessment technique, professional nurses should evaluate it in relation to the performance criteria and the needs of the client group.

Nursing models as a structural framework for assessment

The Roper model will be used to provide the framework for discussing the assessment methods used in nursing (Roper, Logan and Tierney, 1980). This model is chosen because it is one of the most familiar to UK nurses, and because it provides a systematic format for describing assessment. Only subjects with a particular relevance to rehabilitation nursing will be covered, as this is intended to be a representative rather than a comprehensive discussion. Readers should consult the original texts and sources before carrying out any unfamiliar assessment routine described here.

Breathing Clients require special attention when spontaneous breathing is absent or at risk following trauma or neurological damage. There is also a special practice of respiratory rehabilitation for clients with chronic respiratory disorders such as asthma, bronchitis and emphysema. Clients with scoliosis or kyphosis might have respiratory difficulties.

Standard assessment techniques include:

- respiration rate, depth and rhythm or pattern including the use of accessory muscles
- gag reflex
- presence and severity of any dyspnoea or cyanosis
- presence of pain during respiration or cough.

There are scales for breathlessness such as the Borg scale, where the client has to score their own perception of breathlessness (Wilson-Barnett and Batehup, 1988). The Borg scale runs from 0 to 10:0 representing no breathlessness, and 10 representing very, very severe breathlessness (see Table 4.1). Clients indicate their perceived level of dyspnoea by pointing to, or marking, the appropriate point on the printed scale (see Table 4.1).

Table 4.1
*Breathlessness scores
for the Borg scale*

0	no breathlessness
0.5	very, very, slight
1	very slight
2	slight
3	moderate
4	somewhat severe
5	severe
6	
7	very severe
8	
9	
10	very, very, severe

The client may have a cough and this should be assessed for type (productive or dry) and severity. Sputum should be examined for food particles, blood or pus and amount, colour, odour and consistency; specimens of sputum may be sent for laboratory testing. Additionally, peak flow and vital capacity tests can be performed at the bedside to monitor respiratory function. Pulse oximetry measures the level of oxygen saturation in the blood. Auscultation will identify filling defects and areas of consolidation in the lungs. Percussion will also identify consolidation or air trapping in asthmatic or emphysemic clients. A respiration rate higher than 24 or less than 8 should be reported.

Case study 4.1
Respiratory assessment in action

> Rick Swan is a large 30 year old man who weighs 80 kg. He had been feeling unwell for several days, complaining of weakness and 'odd' sensations. He was admitted to the acute admission ward in a busy district general hospital where a tentative diagnosis of Guillain Barré syndrome was made, before he was transferred to the neurology and rehabilitation ward. On admission, he was very anxious and had difficulty with his attention span. He started an intravenous infusion with immunoglobulin when he arrived on the ward. He had half-hourly vital capacity readings because of the danger of loss of respiratory muscle function. Although there was a decline in the readings, they did not reach the level where ventilation was necessary (at approximately 15 ml per kilogram of body weight). His respiration rate was also monitored because an increase in rate may be associated with a decrease in oxygenation. In Rick's case, this level would have been 1.2 L. If this level had been reached, ventilation would have been necessary. Pulse oximetry showed oxygen saturation at no less than 95% each time it was recorded.

Body temperature

Natural temperature of the body may be compromised in neurological damage, especially when the hypothalamus is damaged. People who are immobile may not generate as much metabolic heat as active mobile people. Temperature may need to be monitored in some clients who have defective homeostatic mechanisms, such as a decreased ability to sweat. The neurological client may react unusually to pyrexial conditions because their normal mechanisms are defective (Leslie, 1987). Standard assessment techniques include temperature measurement using a thermometer. A mercury thermometer is still the most widely used instrument, although electronic digital thermometers and disposable strips based on colour changes in indicator chemicals are available. Electronic and tympanic membrane thermometry are particularly useful when the client has uncontrolled body movements as they are quick and avoid the risk of mercury spills. Mercury thermometers are associated with health and safety risks to both staff and clients.

Eating and drinking   Rehabilitation clients may have many problems with eating and drinking. At meal times, the first problem encountered is getting food to the mouth. Paralysis, poor coordination and tremor may all affect intake of nutrients. The control of the muscles of the lips, tongue, cheeks and pharynx may be affected, leading to dysphagia. Impaired sensation from these structures may also cause dysphagia and appetite changes. Cognitive deficits may affect eating and drinking, and malnutrition, over-eating and anorexia (not anorexia nervosa) are fairly common. Assessment techniques depend on the specific problems. Coordination, muscle strength and movement are assessed. This may involve assessing using assistive devices. Dysphagia assessment is complex and will be described separately in 'Problem-related Assessment'. Some health authorities and trusts have an established protocol for swallowing assessment.

Nutritional assessment involves:

- food and fluid balance charts
- blood chemistry (especially nutrient levels)
- weight, body mass index (BMI)
- muscle mass and limb girth measures
- skin-fold thickness
- urinalysis for presence of ketones, nitrogen and calcium loss.

The reliability of some of these tests has been questioned in rehabilitation clients because of the special conditions that may pertain. For instance, BMI has limited value where muscle atrophy is present, which is common in long-term and neurological disability. A person with bilateral leg amputation will have a highly 'abnormal' BMI when compared to a person with legs, but may well have a 'normal' body weight without nutritional implications. The BMI may be calculated by dividing the weight in kilograms by the height in metres squared ($kg/m^2 = BMI$). If the height of a client cannot be measured, or is not known from the client's history, the demispan is an alternative. The distance from the xiphoid process of the sternum to the tip of the outstretched index finger is known as the demispan. Ready reckoner tables are available for calculating BMI using either height or demispan.

Table 4.2
BMI classification

kg/m²	Classification
less than 20	underweight
20–24.9	desirable weight
25–29.9	overweight
30–40	obese
Over 40	morbid obesity

Because of limited usefulness of BMI in some cases, mid upper-arm muscle circumference (MAMC) is used to estimate loss of muscle mass (Bronstein, Popovich and Stewart-Amidei, 1991). To calculate this, the skin-fold thickness (SFT), a measure of subcutaneous fat, is recorded and multiplied by the value of π (3.14), because the arm is a cylinder. The mid upper-arm circumference (MUAC) is then subtracted from this figure: (SFT **2** 3.14) – MUAC = mean upper-arm muscle circumference.

Decreases in this measure show loss of muscle mass. Both the skin-fold thickness and the mid upper-arm circumference are measured at a point over the triceps muscle halfway between the acromion process of the scapula and the olecranon process of the ulna.

The usual measure of hydration is by estimating tissue turgor, by loosely pinching the skin and observing whether it falls back quickly or remains pinched, which indicates relative dehydration. Fluid balance recording will also show if dehydration is an ongoing problem.

Pre-existing food preferences and cultural dietary requirements will have to be recorded as a client with aphasia, for example, may not be able to protest if the wrong food is offered. Cognitive assessment techniques will be discussed separately below but are of importance, because impaired cognition may lead to appetite change.

Elimination   Neurological damage and spinal injuries may lead to loss of conscious control of bowel and bladder. There is a high incidence of continence problems within rehabilitation practice (Charbonneau-Smith, 1993; Gross, 1992). Faecal incontinence and constipation with or without spurious diarrhoea are also common in people with reduced mobility or a neurological diagnosis (Andrews and Greenwood, 1993). Parks lists common bowel problems (1980). The client's medication may have an effect on continence and some of these effects are listed in Smith (1997). Drugs such as oxybutynin, given to improve control of bladder in clients with an unstable neurogenic bladder, may cause constipation or even intestinal obstruction, due to its effects on smooth muscle.

Continence assessment methods include:

- recording a continence history
- keeping a record of bowel and bladder activity such as continence charts or a fluid balance chart to identify patterns
- physical examination including sacral reflexes to establish patho-physiological causes and prognosis (essential)
- urodynamics and ultrasound to diagnose the precise nature of the bladder dysfunction
- rectal examination reveals impaction, which can affect urinary continence, and prostatic enlargement in men.

Mobility factors and manual dexterity must also be taken into account when assessing continence as toileting may be problematic, so functional assessment is part of the test battery for elimination. The environment is included in order to identify access problems. Social factors are important as micturition and defaecation are body functions strongly related to embarrassment and dignity. Cognitive deficits may also cause difficulties, so must be assessed.

Skin   Immobile clients are generally identified as at risk from pressure ulcers. Neurological impairment may increase the risk, if sensation is poor or absent, and loss of continence may compound the risk. Pressure ulcers are not the only skin problem of note: clients with Parkinson's disease may be sweaty (Ross and Crabbe, 1987) and people being treated with corticosteroids may have thin, friable skin. Observation of the skin type is one of the key tasks when assessing the skin. Observation and the use of a pressure sore risk scale is the usual means of assessment. There are several available, but the Braden scale is widely acknowledged as valid and reliable, and was devised for rehabilitation use (Hamilton, 1992). There are standard grading scales of existing pressure ulcers such as the Stirling pressure sore severity scale (Reid and Morison, 1994). In the Stirling scale, ulcers are graded from 0 to 4 (see Table 4.3).

Table 4.3
The Stirling scale for pressure ulcers

0	no clinical evidence of pressure ulcers
1	non-blanchable erythema
2	partial thickness ulcer (epidermis or dermis)
3	full thickness ulcer involving muscle fascia, necrosis may or may not be present
4	a full thickness ulcer involving damage to muscle and down to bone, undermining of edges and sinus formation

If there is a pre-existing pressure sore it may be measured, photographed and depth- or volume-calculated to monitor the progress. Physical examination is also a useful technique in assessing skin integrity, because colour changes are often easy to recognise and occur early in the development of pressure ulcers. The assessment of oral mucous membranes and eye surface is important in some clients with neurological deficits and following the use of some drugs. Poor mouth condition may impair communication.

Mobility   Loss of movement can interfere with many activities of living, and the ability to move about it one of the most importing things in life. Neurological damage, orthopaedic disorders, rhematic disorders and diseases of the cardiovascular and respiratory systems can seriously affect mobility. Assessment of mobility may be complex because mobility is made up of so many subsystems such as sensation, motor nerve action, balance, posture, reflexes and maintaining coordination throughout a movement so that it is performed smoothly and efficiently. Problems may be found in specific joints or limbs that contribute to overall mobility impairment. All these subsystems of movement have to be assessed in order to give an accurate picture of the patient.

Assessment methods of mobility include:

- range of movement (contractures and spasticity)
- muscle strength (asthenia and paresis)
- muscle tone (spasticity and flaccidity)
- balance
- reflexes (hyperreflexia and hyporeflexia)
- gait analysis (ataxia, paralysis, paresis, contractures, spasticity)
- functional assessment (mobility and movement in context)
- sensory assessment (coordination, proprioception and feedback).

Electromyography may be performed if equipment is available. Loss of range of movement of a joint due to contractures is a problem of immobility if not dealt with promptly. There is a contracture assessment scale available (Chraska, Bertolin and Van Dyke, 1994). The scoring is from 0 to 12: 0 to 3 representing no contraction or mild risk; 4 to 7 representing mild contracture; 8 to 10 representing moderate contracture; above ten represents severe contracture. The four areas assessed are pain, function, range of movement (ROM) and nursing care (see Table 4.4) and the scores are totalled to give the contracture risk score.

Table 4.4
Contracture assessment scale

Area	Severe (3)	Moderate (2)	Mild (1)	None (0)
Pain	Pain most of the time, with or without movement. Overt facial signs of pain Guarding while performing passive ROM exercises. Analgesia may not relieve.	Pain with passive ROM exercises. Sometimes pain at rest, relieved by analgesic.	Pain at end of range of passive ROM exercises, resolved by rest. Activity may be slowed. Analgesia not usually required.	Occasional or no pain.

Table 4.4 (contd)

Function	No function possibly due to lack of innervation or fixed nature of the contracture. No active or purposeful movement.	Limited function. Poor coordination due to limited movement. Random joint movements may be present. Limited grasp and release but no strength.	Independent function possible. Gross movements are easy, finer movements may be difficult. Some incoordination may be present. Movements may be uncoordinated. Adaptive devices may be used.	Independent function without assistive devices. Fine movement unimpaired.
Ease of Movement	Fixed joints or limbs. Passive range of movement absent or very limited (less than 25%).	Some passive joint movement (up to 50%). May or may not be able to initiate movement. Joint returns to contracted position.	Nearly full range of passive movement. Some resistance at the end of the range.	Full range of active movement.
Nursing	Very difficult to clean skin and to prevent breakdown. Nail cutting impossible. Skin may be macerated.	Difficult to complete skin care and reposition after care. Odour may be present.	Skin care is easy. Limited ability to reposition.	Easy to clean skin and to reposition after care.

Each joint is assessed separately to give a picture of the client's movement ability. There are standard tables of normal range of movement for joints available in text books and physiotherapy manuals. The physical appearance of the limbs and joints will identify some problems. Spasticity is a problem that affects many patients following stroke or head injury. The modified Ashworth scale (see Table 4.5) is used to grade spasticity (McGuire and Rymer, 1996).

Table 4.5
The modified Ashworth scale for spasticity

0	no increase in muscle tone
1	slight increase in tone (catch and release)
2	slight increase in tone (catch and resistance through less than half of the range of movement)
3	marked increase in tone through most of range of movement
4	considerable increase in tone (passive range of movement difficult)
5	rigidity (flexion or extension) of affected part

Painful shoulder is quite common in stroke as well as joint pains in arthritis, therefore pain assessment is a valuable measure in mobility assessment. Chiropody referral should not be forgotten as poor foot condition contributes to mobility impairment. Assistive devices, such as wheelchairs or frames, are often prescribed to improve mobility and assessment involves use of these.

Rest and sleep

Disorders of sleep patterns occur following many neurological insults and are often reported after head injuries (Giles and Clark-Wilson, 1993). Impaired mobility and reduced sensation may alter the activity level and affect sleep (Andrews and Greenwood, 1993). Loss of sleep is reported as a problem by many people, even in full health. Assessment revolves around close observation of clients and asking them to report on their sleep and levels of fatigue. Fatigue is commonly reported as a symptom of some chronic conditions. The timing and possible causes of fatigue should be noted as part of the overall assessment. A sleep history is carried out as the client may have had an unusual pattern of sleep previously. In some people, routine is important and in order for sleep to occur, the routine needs to be followed. This can be established during a sleep history. The other factor in sleep assessment is the environment; the nurse should not only look at the clients and their history but also at the present environment, to ensure that the conditions for sleep are optimal. Instrumental observation is possible, for example, with electroencephalography, or compact body-worn monitoring devices that record movement over a 24-hour period, can demonstrate patterns in sleep. This may be particularly useful when the client has an altered (or suspected altered) conscious state.

Communication

The simplified view of communication in Box 4.5 identifies a number of areas in which a message being sent can be disrupted. It has three levels, linguistic, physiological and acoustic. Cortical lesions may disrupt the source of the message (expressive dysphasia), or its interpretation (receptive dysphasia), or both (global dysphasia). Interruption to the motor control of the mouth can cause dysarthria, motor deficits in the upper limbs will cause an analogous problem with signing or writing. Deafness or visual loss can interfere with reception of the message. Assessment aims to identify these problems, which may be concurrent, and where necessary, separate them from non-language problems. Cognitive deficits, confusion or dementia may mimic a communication problem.

Box 4.5
The communication chain

- Source of the message (the cerebral cortex and motor pathways)
- Transmitter (the vocal tract for speech, gestural system for deaf signing, or hand movements for writing)
- Receiver (the ears and eyes)
- Interpreting system (the cerebral cortex and auditory pathways)
(Denes and Pinson, 1993)

Assessment methods are usually carried out by speech and language therapists but a number of observational techniques are available for basic assessment by nurses. These are based around the client's response to a specified task. For example, to test understanding of speech, asking the client to carry out some motor task that is within their functional capability. It is important not to give clues by other means such as gesture if the nurse is to assess only the understanding of language. Sometimes this understanding can be further tested by asking the client to do one task, say brushing the teeth, and demonstrating another, such as putting on spectacles. If this incongruity produces confusion in the client, understanding of language is probably intact. The production of speech is assessed by asking the client to tell something, perhaps their address. Ideally this should be verifiable. Listening to the meaning and articulation of their reply will inform the assessment.

Reading and writing may be tested simply, by asking the client to perform these activities. If speech is impaired or absent, reading can be assessed by writing a request for some identifiable action, such as sticking out the tongue, and noting if the client performs the requested action. Writing may be affected by motor impairment. More detailed tests used by the rehabilitation team include the Boston VAMC communication assessment tool (Shanks, 1983) which tests:

- level of information processing and orientation
- reading comprehension relative to speech comprehension
- ability to follow commands.

These give the team the opportunity to analyse the communication deficit and select an appropriate treatment regime. The discussion has concentrated on verbal expression (that is, use of language in all its forms) but non-verbal communication via facial expression and body language should also be assessed where necessary.

Sexuality Many rehabilitation clients, by the nature of their diagnosis, may have impaired sexual function. This may be due to loss of mobility, pain or decreased or increased libido. Sexual expression is a personal and emotive thing and nurses and clients may choose to ignore it. However, the issues must be addressed if the client is to achieve optimum independence. The gender of the assessing nurse may be very important for the client. If the cognitive processes are affected, there may be issues concerned with consent. Assessment is based around a sexual history and physical examination methods such as mobility, sensation and sexual function. There is more to sexual assessment than the physical aspects. The PLISSIT model (Permission, Limited Information, Specific Suggestion and Intensive Therapy) provides a framework for assessing the patient (Annon and Robinson, 1978). The client needs permission to talk about and take part in sexual activity. There are several myths around sex and people with disabilities which need to be dealt with, such as the appropriateness of sex and some sexual practices that might not have been considered premorbidly. The nurse can start the assessment process by giving the permission, which is the first level of intervention in the PLISSIT model.

Questions that might be included in a sexuality assessment include (Schepp, 1986):

1. Level of sex education
2. How disability and illness affect the sexual functioning
3. How the client assesses the functioning of their own sexual organs
4. Fertility, family and marriage issues
5. What treatments are planned or in progress
6. Body image, masculinity and femininity
7. Communication
8. Myths about sexuality and interpersonal relationships
9. Does the patient consider themselves celibate? Sexual orientation?
10. Social and sexual skills to facilitate sexual satisfaction
11. History of rape, abuse or trauma
12. Level of sexual interest
13. Level of acceptance of illness and relationship of this to sexuality.

Certain drugs will affect sexual function and a full history will need to include drug history. The current edition of British National Formulary lists side-effects of drugs that may affect sexual function (Joint Formulary Committee, 1998). Continence is important in the expression of sexuality because of the close anatomical relationship of the urinary tract and the genitalia. Otherwise normal sexual function may be prevented simply by incontinence or fear of it. Sexuality is often taken to include body image issues, as they may be related to sexual attractiveness and therefore confidence and esteem.

Work and leisure

The client needs to work or have leisure activities in order to maintain self esteem and creative expression. Mobility, movement and sensory loss may impede both work and leisure activities. Loss of cognitive function will certainly affect the client's ability to enjoy and perform work and leisure activities. Assessment methods are based around functional assessment and mobility (see above). Another important aspect of work and leisure assessment is the client's sensory ability, perception and cognitive issues such as concentration, depression, memory and neglect.

Hygiene and grooming

These interrelated aspects of daily life depend on the client's ability to be able to complete purposeful movements, sensory ability, perception, and cognitive issues such as concentration, memory and neglect. Specific problems may be related to the inability to reach lower parts of the trunk and legs due to loss of flexibility or mobility. These areas include, of course, the perineum and genitalia which may need special attention if the client is incontinent. Foot and nail care are important, especially in people who still have some residual mobility, and in diabetic patients. Assessment is usually functional, highlighting upper limb movement and control. Observation of skin and checking pressure areas and feet is also necessary. Hair, nails, eyes and mouth will need to be included in the overall hygiene and grooming observations. Cognitive and sensory assessment methods are to be included because the client's appearance may depend on these being intact. For example, clients with neglect may not arrange their hair or apply make-up according to usual conventions, resulting in a strange appearance. Behavioural problems may lead to inability to recognise, or refusal to acknowledge, a hygiene need.

Coping

Rehabilitation clients will probably have a range of emotional and behavioural reactions to their change of health and ability status. In neurological disorders, behaviour may be affected so that the response is abnormal. It may be absent, prolonged or inappropriate. Clients with chronic illness are fearful of loss of function or body parts (Strain, 1979). Following loss of function, the client may go through a classical grieving process (Kübler-Ross, 1969). Nurses need to assess the stage of the grieving process so that the appropriate interventions can be offered. Assessment is complex and is based on history and analysis of coping behaviours from the client and family. Specific assessment scales exist for depression and anxiety and family function. These test scales may be administered by a clinical psychologist or occupational therapist, but the results are relevant to nursing assessment and the subsequent care planning.

In all nursing models, it is essential to ascertain the level of independence of the patient. In acute stages, the nurse may have to provide all the care necessary, but in many instances, even in acute illness, clients may be able to contribute greatly to their own care. This level of care is included in the initial assessment. The object in rehabilitation is usually to withdraw as much nursing assistance as possible and let the client achieve maximum control and participation.

Case study 4.2
Assessment on admission

Neil Butler is a man aged 19. He has been admitted to the rehabilitation unit from a neurosurgery ward following a road traffic accident where he sustained head injury. He was deeply unconscious with a Glasgow coma score of 8. After a craniotomy and evacuation of a blood clot, he made slow progress and is now conscious. He has dysarthria and dysphagia and he is losing weight. He has a spastic paralysis of his legs and poor control of his arms and hands. Before his accident, he was an engineering student at university and was described by his friends as 'happy-go-lucky'.

On admission, he was accompanied by his parents. The staff on the unit established the following items for priority of assessment. More in-depth assessment was carried out during the first 3 weeks following admission.

- **Weight loss**. Body mass index and mean upper arm muscle mass were calculated. Weekly weighing was ordered. These can be compared with normal values to identify the nutritional needs.
- **Mobility**. Neil was assessed by the physiotherapist because of the spastic paralysis and the need to initiate treatment plan quickly to prevent establishment of abnormal movement patterns.
- **Dysarthria**. The speech and language therapist confirmed the diagnosis and planned treatment to improve his breath control and articulatory gestures.
- **Dysphagia**. Neil was seen by the speech therapist for a swallowing assessment. It was decided to create a temporary gastrostomy to deliver most of the nutrition, but small amounts were still given by mouth.
- **Functional assessment**. An occupational therapist assessed Neil using the Barthel activities of daily living index (see below). Four days after admission, his score was zero.
- **Bowel and bladder**. A record was kept of incidences of incontinence so that any underlying pattern could be discovered. He was checked hourly and the result recorded for faecal and urinary incontinence.

■ **Psychological profile**. The clinical psychologist on the unit assessed Neil to identify any cognitive deficits. He was found to have a poor attention span and long-term memory loss. His poor speech and mobility led to expression of emotion and frustration as outbursts of shouting.

■ **General medical examination**. This did not reveal any special problems that were not identified on other assessment tests. He had no visual or hearing impairment.

■ **Family**. His parents were interviewed over several days. They are both middle-aged professional people in full-time employment. They decided to take Neil home: there is a room on the ground floor of the house that can be converted for easy access. They are concerned about his outbursts and their finances because one of them may have to give up work to look after Neil. Neil has an older married sister with a young child, and a brother of 17. The younger brother is at sixth form college studying for A levels. His college work has been deteriorating since the accident.

Specific assessment measures

Functional assessment

The notion of functional assessment is fundamental in rehabilitation practice. In order to carry out every-day activities, a wide variety of sensory, perceptual and motor skills are necessary. Several tests have been devised to provide an objective scale which assesses a client's ability to perform these functions, hence functional assessment. A widely used scale is the Barthel activities of daily living index (Mahoney and Barthel, 1965). Originally, this consisted of a 100-point scale, but more recent versions of the Barthel index score 0, 1, 2 or 3 to give a total of 20 points. Clients are assessed according to ten key activities (see Box 4.6).

Box 4.6
Barthel index scoring system

Bowels	0 = depends on intervention
	1 = some episodes of soiling
	2 = continent
Bladder	0 = depends on intervention
	1 = some episodes of soiling
	2 = continent
Grooming	0 = dependent
	1 = independent
Toiletting	0 = dependent
	1 = assistance required
	2 = independent

Feeding	0 = dependent
	1 = assistance required
	2 = independent
Transfer	0 = dependent
	1 = maximal assistance
	2 = minimal assistance
	3 = independent
Mobility	0 = dependent
	1 = independent with wheelchair
	2 = assistance from another person to walk
	3 = independent
Dressing	0 = dependent
	1 = assistance required
	2 = independent
Stairs	0 = dependent
	1 = assistance required
	2 = independent
Bathing	0 = dependent
	1 = independent

(Mahoney and Barthel, 1965)

Box 4.7
Functional indepen-dence measure (FIM) activities

Self care	Feeding
	Grooming
	Bathing
	Dressing upper body
	Dressing lower body
	Toileting
Sphincter control	Bladder
	Bowel
Mobility	Transferring bed, chair or wheelchair
	Transferring toilet
	Transferring bath and shower
Locomotion	Ambulation
	Stairs
Communication	Comprehension
	Expression
Social cognition	Social interaction
	Problem solving
	Memory

(Granger, Hamilton and Sherwin, 1986)

Older versions had weightings of 0, 5, 10 and sometimes 15, giving a total of 100 possible points. The smaller total of 20 gives a more manageable and less inflated score. Although the index is fairly old, dating back into the 1960s, new versions are still appearing and it is widely used because of its simplicity. It serves as a sort of gold standard of functional assessment scales. One criticism is that it does not include any items which assess the cognitive, communicative and emotional aspects of functional activity. These items have to be estimated by separate techniques.

Other scales have been devised to give precise detail and include other items for assessment. A widely-used scale is the functional independence measure (FIM) (Granger, Hamilton and Sherwin, 1986). This scale has 18 key activities, listed in Box 4.7.

There are four categories and seven points in the scoring system for FIM (see Table 4.6).

Table 4.6
Scoring system for the functional independence measure

Category	Score	Level of independence
Independence	7	Complete independence. Action performed safely and in a reasonable time
Modified independence	6	Aids are required but no human assistance is needed. More time may be taken or safety issues may be involved
Modified dependence	5	Supervision required, or cueing
	4	Minimal assistance required, the patient performs 75% or more of the task
	3	Moderate assistance required, the patient performs 50% to 74% of the task
Complete dependence	2	Maximal assistance required, the patient performs 25% to 49% of the task
	1	Total assistance, the patient performs less than 25% of the task

The scoring is precisely specified. To ensure reliability, there is a 'credentialing' program designed to give practitioners the skill to produce repeatable, consistent results. The FIM scale has communication and social cognition items included. The Barthel index and FIM do not measure precisely the same variables.

Case study 4.3
Using functional assessment

Katie Seymour is a 75 year old woman. She had a stroke 7 weeks ago and has been transferred to the rehabilitation unit for assessment and an intensive program before she can go home.

Self-care

Feeding: Mrs Seymour can feed herself provided she has a thick-handled fork and a plate with a guard. The food has to be cut up. She takes a longer time than most clients to feed herself. There is a slight risk of choking as she is mildly dysphagic.

(Score 4)

Grooming: Mrs Seymour can comb her own hair with a specially adapted comb with a large grip. She can remove but cannot clean her dentures as she has a weak right arm and cannot grip them for brushing. She cannot apply her own make up. She can wash and dry her hands slowly.

(Score 3)

Bathing: She cannot bathe herself. She needs help getting into the bath and cannot reach all skin areas for washing and drying.

(Score 2)

Dressing upper body: Mrs Seymour can put on outer garments but needs help with buttons and fastenings.

(Score 4)

Dressing lower body: She cannot dress her lower half and needs maximal help. She can move to assist dressing.

(Score 2)

Toiletting: She cannot remove her clothes but she can transfer with help. She cannot use toilet paper.

(Score 2)

Sphincter control

Bladder: Mrs Seymour has got some control and can ask to go to the toilet but needs help in the toilet. She also has accidents and wears a pad.

(Score 3)

Bowel: Mrs Seymour has got some control and asks to go to the toilet where she needs help. She is often constipated and requires suppositories. Soiling accidents happen occasionally.

(Score 3)

Mobility

Transferring to bed, chair or wheelchair: She can stand with assistance and transfer from bed to chair and back.

(Score 4)

Transferring to toilet: Mrs Seymour can transfer with assistance to stand and remove clothing.

(Score 4)

Transferring to bath and shower: She requires maximal assistance to get in and out of the bath.

(Score 2)

Locomotion
Ambulation: Mrs Seymour cannot move more than a few feet in a self-propelled chair. (She is to be assessed for an electrically-powered chair soon.)

(Score 2)

Stairs: Mrs Seymour cannot manage stairs at all.

(Score 1)

Communication
Comprehension: Mrs Seymour has good comprehension and follows spoken and written commands.

(Score 7)

Expression: She can express complex ideas with some difficulty, words are not always clear and she has difficulty finding the right words, but nevertheless can communicate.

(Score 6)

Social Cognition
Social interaction: Mrs Seymour participates well with staff and family, but unfamiliar situations confuse her.

(Score 6)

Problem-solving: She has some difficulty in performing tasks and does not always perform complex actions correctly.

(Score 6)

Memory: Mrs Seymour recognises people and situations but needs prompting for some therapeutic activities and hospital routines.

(Score 6)

Mrs Seymour's motor subscore is 36 and her cognitive subscore is 31 giving a total of 67 (A total of 119 points is available on FIM).

Mrs Seymour would have scored 5 using the Barthel index. The FIM motor subscore gives her a score of 51% of the total on items equivalent to the Barthel index. The Barthel percentage is 25%. FIM is more sensitive because it has a wider scoring range, making it more able to detect smaller residual amounts of functional ability.

FIM is not suitable for children because of the special developmental aspects of functional assessment. A version has been specially devised for use with children, called WeeFim. Criticism of FIM includes the relative shortage of items assessing psychosocial aspects. This has lead to another scale, the functional assessment measure (FAM) which includes more items than FIM although the scoring is essentially the same. All the FIM items are included, but FAM additionally contains the items in Box 4.8.

Box 4.8
Functional assess-
ment measure (FAM)
added items

Self care	Swallowing
Mobility	Transfer to car
Locomotion	Community mobility
Communication	Reading
	Writing
	Speech intelligibility
Psychological adjustment	Emotional status
	Adjustment to limitation
	Employability
Cognitive function	Orientation
	Attention
	Safety judgement

It can be seen that new categories of psychological function and cognitive function replace the FIM category 'social cognition'. FAM therefore contains a total of 30 assessed items. In both FIM and FAM, 'not applicable' is not accepted and the scorer must enter a score of 1 if not applicable would be chosen or the item is considered too risky to assess. The assessments for FIM and FAM are usually made by direct observation by members of the rehabilitation team.

There are many other functional assessment scales available. Derick Wade includes many others in his book (1992), which should be consulted for a full account. Sometimes used in the USA are:

■ The PULSES Profile. PULSES is an acronym standing for physical condition, upper extremities, lower extremities, sensory components, excretory function and mental and emotion status. The profile gives a score from 1 to 4 (1 representing no abnormality and 4 representing severe abnormalities). PULSES is not a scale and there is a separate score for each of the subsections (Granger and Gresham, 1984).
■ PECS is an acronym for patient evaluation and conference systems. In PECS, members of the interdisciplinary team carry out their own professional assessment which is then put together to form a comprehensive evaluation of the client's condition. Test items cover activities of daily living, nursing, mobility, communication, aids and devices, occupation, medical assessment and medication, nutrition, social interactions, psychology, pain, respiratory function, nutrition and leisure activities (Harvey and Jellinek, 1981).
■ Katz index of independence in ADL. Six categories – bathing, dressing, toiletting, transferring, continence and feeding – are

assessed on a three-point scale of independent, assisted, or dependent (Katz, Ford and Moskowitz, 1963).

Other functional assessment measures used in the UK are:

- Nottingham 10-point ADL index. A simple measure where ten items are scored 0 or 1. The patient receives a 1 for each item they can do. The ten items are drink from a cup, eat, wash face and hands, transfer from bed to chair, walk around house, use toilet, dress, undress, make a hot drink, have a bath. The score is simply added up to give the index (Wade, 1992).
- Rivermead activities of daily living scales. The patient is assessed on a 2-point scale of 1 for independence and 0 for dependence. There are two categories of items, self-care (16 items) and household (15 items) (Wade, 1992).

Problem-related assessment

Swallowing and dysphagia

Swallowing difficulty is relatively common in neurological rehabilitation. Most clients with a speech or language problem may be at risk of dysphagia because the muscles of speech are primarily the muscles of eating and swallowing. This is the original function because eating and swallowing predate the evolution of speech by countless ages (Aitchison, 1996). If the muscles of speech cannot be controlled to produce accurate speech sounds, then swallowing may also be impaired by the same lack of control. In many places, the speech and language therapist (SLT) will make the detailed swallowing assessment because of their specific training in the control of mouth movements. However, nurses may need to make their own assessment before the arrival of the SLT. Some hospitals provide a swallowing assessment protocol to screen the clients who need urgent referral from those where no special referral is needed. Table 4.7 is

Table 4.7
Julia Farr Centre swallowing assessment protocol (adapted from Russell and Hill, 1992)

Assess swallowing of	Outcome	Action
Saliva	Swallows saliva without problems	Assess swallowing water
	Has difficulties in swallowing saliva	Perform detailed eating assessment or refer to speech and language therapist.
Water and fluids	Manages fluids without difficulty	Assess with puree or thickened fluids
	Has difficulties swallowing fluids	Perform detailed eating assessment or refer to speech and language therapist.

Table 4.7 (cont'd)

Pureed diet or thick-ened fluids	Swallows puree with no difficulty	Assess with minced diet
	Has difficulty swallowing pureed food or thickened fluid	Perform detailed eating assessment or refer to SLT.
Minced Diet	Has no difficulties with minced texture	Assess with solid food
	Has difficulty swallowing minced texture	Perform detailed eating assessment or refer to SLT.
Solid food	Has no difficulty with solid food	Safe to give full diet but continue to observe the patient at mealtimes.
	Cannot manage solid diet	Perform detailed eating assessment or refer to SLT.

an example of swallowing assessment protocol based on the assessment model from the Julia Farr Centre in Australia.

Detailed swallowing assessment needs to include:

- cognitive problems
- oral preparatory phase of swallowing (lip closure and chewing)
- oral phase of swallowing (formation of the bolus and movement of the tongue)
- pharyngeal phase (closure of the nasal cavity, elevation of the larynx, epiglottis, closure of the laryngeal aditus by the epiglottis)
- oesophageal phase (peristalsis conveys bolus down oesophagus)
- timing of the swallow
- modifications to food and fluid texture
- nutritional assessment.

It is important to state the position of the gag reflex in swallowing assessment. While the gag reflex may form part of the assessment because it reveals information about the cranial nerve, it does not predict safe or unsafe swallowing. People without neurological problems may not have a gag reflex, especially elderly people (Davies et al., 1995). In other words, many people swallow safely without the gag reflex and others may have difficulty swallowing with an intact gag reflex. The cough reflex, however, is protective, and indicates the client's ability to protect their own airway.

There are other forms of assessment that can be used to assess the swallow. Videofluoroscopy enables the therapists to see into the pharynx and larynx in a non-invasive way. Pooling of food and fluids in the valleculae after completion of the swallow indicates a particular risk of aspiration. Indirect laryngoscopy using a laryngeal mirror may be useful. A fine fibreoptic endoscope can be passed nasally, so that direct visualisation of the pharynx is possible. The quality of the voice is of great importance in swallowing assessment. Speech with air leaking through the nasal cavity (hypernasality), due to poor or absent closure of the velum against the posterior pharyngeal wall, may precede nasal regurgitation or aspiration. A hyponasal voice, one usually described as 'nasal' (as in a cold, but a misnomer because the so-called nasal voice of a cold has no nasal resonance!) suggests occlusion of the nasal passages (Miller, 1992). A 'wet, gurgly' voice may indicate mucus production in the inflamed larynx following repeated aspiration episodes.

Pain Pain is a frequent problem in rehabilitation. It occurs in patients with neurological and rheumatological diagnoses and many others. Acute pain and cancer pain are the subjects of a wide range of publications. Management of these forms of pain may be well documented and therapeutic regimes are widely practised. Chronic pain has gone beyond the normal protective and warning function and gathers up with it a collection of physical, psychological and social components (Bowman, 1994). Careful assessment is very important if the patient is to obtain relief from the pain. Pain may also prevent full participation in the rehabilitation program, therefore pain control becomes a prime objective. The following effects are related to chronic pain (Simon, 1996):

- adaptation to sympathetic nervous system arousal
- deconditioning and inactivity leading to impaired function
- depression
- family relationships are affected
- sexual relationships are affected
- dependence on analgesics
- sleep is affected.
- weight gain
- passivity and dependence as part of coping
- attention and support for being in pain are provided by the family
- occupational disruption and financial disruption.

In rehabilitation practice, pain is commonly reported in multiple sclerosis and stroke (both neurogenic pain and shoulder pain). Phantom limb pain affects clients following amputation and stroke and spinal injury, although in this case the limb still exists, although the neurological connection has been severed. It goes without saying that pain is one of the symptoms that people fear most, and it must be addressed. There are a number of pain assessment methods. The McGill pain inventory, where the patient is scored on several items, includes sensory, affective and evaluative aspects of pain. There is also a numerical scale and a body diagram to indicate the location of the pain. Pain intensity scales are commonly used and consist of a line that may have adjective descriptions of the pain, for example, no pain, slight, moderate, severe and very severe. Other scales use numbers and the client selects the actual rating, and yet others offer no intermediate points between pain free and severe pain: the patient indicates with a cross. In rehabilitation settings, the assessment methods selected should adequately reflect the emotional and psychosocial components of the pain.

Sensory assessment

The sensory division of the nervous system consists of organs of special sense such as vision, hearing, taste and smell and general sense such as, heat, vibration, touch and so on. Sensation provides information about the internal and external environments. The reaction of the body to change depends on sensory input. Therefore reactions, including protective reflexes, normal movement and even metabolic responses may be profoundly affected in sensory loss. Movement is so dependent on sensory input that the client with diminished or absent balance and proprioception may be unable to achieve mobility. There is also an aesthetic component to sensation, therefore vision, hearing and taste are especially highly prized. These aesthetic qualities include appreciation of music, natural beauty and colour and the enjoyment of food. For the client to function optimally it is essential for sensation to be included in routine assessment. Routine assessment of sensation must include:

- sight
- hearing
- smell
- taste
- proprioception
- touch
- vibration
- heat.

The perception (that is, the interpretation of sensation) should also be assessed, because disordered perception is common following neurological damage. Disorders include neglect or inattention, hemianopia, and the various agnosias.

Cognitive assessment

A large part of the rehabilitation program for a neurological client may consist of dealing with cognitive problems. Some of these are dealt with in general terms by functional assessment (where cognition is assessed as part of function), but there is also a need for more specific cognitive assessment. The Good Samaritan Hospital in Washington State, USA, have a battery of cognitive tests based on the hospital's process-specific approach to cognitive rehabilitation. These tests include the following elements of cognitive function:

- attention and concentration
- orientation
- memory
- visuo-spatial processing
- reasoning/concept formation
- motor planning
- executive function.

These areas of cognition are all assessed on a 6-point scale. The assessor chooses a level which best describes the client's level. Each of the scale levels consists of a series of statements describing the cognitive conditions at that level. The descriptors are precisely detailed to provide reliability. Derick Wade describes several individual tests of cognitive function in his book (Wade, 1992).

Anxiety and depression

Anxiety and depression are two problems commonly perceived for a rehabilitation client adjusting to a new level of functional and cognitive ability. Psychiatric referral may be necessary in some cases where these reach pathological proportions. A common assessment scale is the hospital anxiety and depression scale (HAD), which is in questionnaire format. The final score indicates the level of the depression and anxiety; two separate items are scored as normal, borderline abnormal or abnormal (that is, requiring treatment). There are other scales in use and these can be found in Derick Wade's book (1992).

Challenging behaviour

Behavioural changes following neurological damage are well known. Anxiety and depression have already been discussed. Other behaviours which may pose a challenge to the rehabilitation team include apathy, poor attention span, aggression and disinhibition. The motivational assessment scale is used for clients with learning difficulties and mental health problems (Durand, 1988). It is designed to identify situations in which a client is likely to exhibit challenging behaviour, and assess the possible reasons for the behaviour. The scale is a questionnaire with 16 items which are scored from zero to 6 points. The ratings are allocated so that the questions are answered from never (0), via half the time (3) to always (6), with intermediate points. The scores are entered on a grid and the columns added to give the relative ranking of four behaviour 'situations'. These are:

- sensory (the need to touch, feel, taste, smell, etc.)
- escape (to avoid activities, people or objects)
- attention (to get the attention of another person)
- tangible (the need to hold, possess or perform activity).

The motivational assessment scale is best used as part of a full assessment of the client. It is not apparent that this test has been widely used in rehabilitation patients.

Family

The role of the family (which for the sake of this discussion is taken to include close friends and other informal care-givers) is fundamental to the rehabilitation process. In fact it has been said that rehabilitation cannot be successful without the cooperation and involvement of the family (Kenney Weeks, 1995). The family, including the client, should be seen as a functional unit with all the members interdependent on each other (Davies, 1988). The Family Coping Index Scoring Profile provides a basis on which the family can be assessed (Freeman, Clark and Lowe, 1964). The family are rated on a 5-point scale for:

- physical independence
- therapeutic independence
- knowledge of condition
- application of principles of general hygiene
- attitudes towards health care
- emotional competence
- family living patterns
- physical environment
- use of community resources.

These nine categories have three levels of descriptive statements numbered 1 (no competence), 3 (moderate competence) and 5 (complete competence). Scorers are able to allocate 2 and 4 value scores at their own discretion. When the assessment is complete, the nurse will have a profile of the family which can provide the basis of planning nursing intervention with them. Other family assessment scales are available and one, the FAMTOOL, has been recently developed. FAMTOOL is a scale that assesses family health. 12 positive statements have four possible responses (0 = false, 1 = mostly false, 3 = mostly true, 4 = true) and scoring is thus from 0 to 36 where 36 indicates high-level family function (Weeks and O'Connor, 1997).

Age-related assessment

Some assessment methods are related to the age of the client. WeeFim is an example that has already been discussed in the section about functional assessment. Another age related system is SCOPE (self care of elder persons evaluation), a method for establishing the self-care status of elderly people (Dellasega and Clark,

1995). SCOPE looks at 13 activities: breathing, eating, bladder control, bowel control, sleeping, mobility, bathing, dressing, grooming, cognition, vision, hearing and social activity. The scoring system is a 0 to 5 scale (0 = no apparent ability for self-care, 1 = minimal ability for self-care, 2 = can perform activity with moderate amount of assistance, 3 = can perform activity with minimal assistance, 4 = can perform the activity with intermittent assistance, 5 = completely independent in self care).

The scores have to be adapted for the sensory social and cognitive items but these follow the basic ideology of the scoring method, for example, a mid score for vision is the use of glasses or other visual aids. The maximum score is 65, which indicates independence. The interpretation of the scale is:

- 50–65 independent
- 40–49 needs minimal assistance and can do most activities of daily living alone
- 25–39 moderate amount of assistance and supervision needed but can still perform some activities alone
- 10–24 able to perform some basic care alone but otherwise needs maximal care
- 0–9 requires total care.

Disease-related assessment

There are several assessment methods that are used for specific diseases. Stroke, multiple sclerosis, Parkinson's disease, head injury and spinal injury have tests to measure the severity or effects of the illness. These tests and rating scales may not be part of nursing practice but nurses may be involved in data collection, as a member of the rehabilitation team, and for supporting the client and family undergoing assessment.

Conclusion

Assessment is the first step in the process for care of clients and their families. It has a role in clinical management, financial and economic planning, research and education.

This chapter has examined the nurse's role in assessment as part of providing nursing care and the nurse's role in the multidisciplinary team. Nurses are autonomous practitioners in their own right, as well as members of the multidisciplinary team. Knowledge of assessment, as part of the process of rehabilitation care, enables nurses to contribute fully.

References

Aitchison, J. (1996) *The Seeds of Speech*. Cambridge: Cambridge University Press.

Andrews, K. & Greenwood, R. (1993) Physical consequences of neurological disablement. In *Neurological Rehabilitation*, Greenwood, R. et al. Edinburgh: Churchill Livingstone.

Annon, J. S. & Robinson, C.H.(1978) The use of vicarious models in treatment of sexual concerns. *Handbook of Sex Therapy*, ed. Lo-Piccolo, J. & LoPiccolo, L. New York: Plenum Press.

Bowman, J.M. (1994) Experiencing the chronic pain phenomenon: a study. *Rehabilitation Nursing*, **19**, 91–95.

Bronstein, K., Popovich, J.M. & Stewart-Amidei, C. (1991) *Promoting Stroke Recovery*. St Louis: Mosby Year Book.

Charbonneau-Smith, R. (1993) No touch catheterization and infection rates in a select spinal cord injury situation. *Rehabilitation Nursing*, **18**, 296–299 & 305.

Chraska, K., Bertolin, B. & Van Dyke, K. (1994) *Rehabilitation Nursing: Course Syllabus*. Puyallup, Washington: Good Samaritan Rehabilitation Center.

Davies, A.E., Kidd, D., Stone, S.P., & MacMahon, J. (1995) Pharyngeal sensation and gag reflex in healthy subjects. *The Lancet*, **345**, 487–488.

Davies, B.M. (1988) Social factors in disability. In *Rehabilitation of the Physically Disabled Adult*, Goodwill, J. & Chamberlain, A. London: Chapman and Hall Medical.

Dellasega, C. & Clark, D. (1995) SCOPE: A practical method for assessing the self care status of elderly persons. *Rehabilitation Nursing Research*, **4**, 128–135.

Denes, P.B. & Pinson, E.N. (1993) *The Speech Chain: the Physics and Biology of Spoken Language*, 2nd edn. New York: W.H. Freeman and Co.

Durand, V.M. (1988) Motivational Assessment Scale. In *Dictionary of Behavioural Assessment Techniques*, ed. Hersen M. & Bellack, A.F. New York: Pergamon Press.

Freeman, R., Clark, M. & Lowe, M. (1964) *The Family Coping Index*. Richmond, Virginia: Richmond Instructive Nurse Association and City Health Department and John Hopkins School of Public Health.

Giles, G.M. & Clark-Wilson, J. (1993) *Brain Injury Rehabilitation: a Neurofunctional Approach*. London: Chapman and Hall.

Gless, P. (1995) Applying the Roy adaptation model to the care of clients with quadriplegia. *Rehabilitation Nursing*, **20**, 11–16.

Granger, C.V. & Gresham, G.E. (1984) *Functional Assessment in Rehabilitation Medicine*. Baltimore: Williams and Wilkins.

Granger, C.V., Hamilton, B.B. & Sherwin, F.S. (1986) *Guide for the Use of the Uniform Data Set for Medical Rehabilitation*. Buffalo, New York: Uniform Data System for Medical Rehabilitation Project Office.

Gresham, G.E., Duncan, P.W., Stason, W.B. (1995) Post-Stroke Rehabilitation: Assessment, Referral and Patient Management. USA: Agency for Health Care Policy and Research.

Gross, J.C. (1992) Bladder dysfunction after stroke. *Urologic Nursing*, **12**, 55–63.

Hamilton, F. (1992) An analysis of the literature pertaining to pressure sore risk-assessment scales. *Journal of Clinical Nursing*, **1**, 185–193.

Harvey, R.F. & Jellinek, H.M. (1981) Functional performance assessment: a program approach. *Archives of Physical Medicine and Rehabilitation*, **62**, 456–460.

Hoeman, S. (1996) *Rehabilitation Nursing: Process and Application*, 2nd edn. St Louis: Mosby.

Joint Formulary Committee (1998) *British National Formulary 30*. London: British Medical Association and Royal Pharmaceutical Society of Great Britain.

Jones, A. (1995) Utilizing Peplau's psychodynamic theory for stroke patient care. *Journal of Clinical Nursing*, **4**, 49–54.

Katz, S., Ford, A.B. & Moskwitz, R.W. (1963) Studies in illness of the aged. The index of ADL: a standardised measure of biological and psychosocial function. JAMA, **185**, 914–919.

Kenney Weeks, S. (1995) What are the educational needs of prospective family caregivers of newly disabled adults. *Rehabilitation Nursing*, **20**, 256–260.

Knust, S.J. & Quarn, J.M. (1983) Integration of the self care theory with rehabilitation nursing. *Rehabilitation Nursing*, **8**, 26–28.

Kübler-Ross, E. (1969) *On Death and Dying*. New York: Macmillan.

Leslie, D.J. (1987) Patient assessment: history taking and physical examination. In *Neurologic Problems*, Peck, V. Springhouse, Pennsylvania: Springhouse Corporation.

Lumley, J.S.P. & Benjamin, W. (1994) *Research: Some Ground Rules*. Oxford: Oxford University Press.

Mahoney, F.I. & Barthel, D.W. (1965) Functional evaluation: the Barthel index. *Maryland State Medical Journal*, **14**, 61–65.

McGuire, J.R. & Rymer, W.Z. (1996) Spasticity: mechanisms and management. In *Medical Management of Long Term Disability*, Green, D. Boston: Butterworth-Heinemann.

Miller, R. (1992) Clinical examination for dysphagia. In *Dysphagia*, ed. Groher, M.E. Boston: Butterworth-Heinemann.

Parks, A.G. (1980) Faecal incontinence. In *Incontinence and its Management*, 2nd edn, ed. Mandelstam, D. London: Croom Helm.

Piazza, D. & Foote, A. (1990) Roy's adaptation model: a guide for rehabilitation nursing practice. *Rehabilitation Nursing*, **15**, 254–259.

Reid, J. & Morison, M. (1994) Towards a consensus: classification of pressure sores. *Journal of Wound Care*, **3**, 157–160.

Roper, N., Logan, W. & Tierney, A. (1980) *Using a Model for Nursing*. Edinburgh: Churchill Livingstone.

Ross, A.P. & Crabbe, R.A. (1987) Degenerative and autoimmune disorders: progressive problems. In *Neurologic Problems*, Peck, V. Springhouse, Pennsylvania: Springhouse Corporation.

Russell, A. & Hill, P. (1992) *Transitional Feeding*. Unley, South Australia: Julia Farr Centre Foundation.

Schepp, K.F. (1986). *Sexual Counselling: a training program*. Accelerated Development Inc: Indiana.

Shanks, S. (1983) *Nursing and the Management of Adult Communication Disorders*. San Diego: College Hill Press.

Simon, J.M. (1996) Chronic pain syndrome: nursing assessment and intervention. *Rehabilitation Nursing*, **21**, 13–18.

Smith, M. (1997) Medication and continence. In *Promoting Continence*, ed. Getliffe, K., & Dolman, M. London: Baillière Tindall.

Strain, J.J. (1979) Psychological reactions to chronic illness. *Psychiatric Quarterly*, 51, 173–181.

Wade, D. (1992) *Measurement in Neurological Rehabilitation*. Oxford: Oxford University Press.

Weeks, S.K. & O'Connor, P.C. (1997) The FAM-TOOL family health assessment tool. *Rehabilitation Nursing*, **22**, 188–191.

Wilson-Barnett, J. & Batehup, L. (1988) *Patient Problems: a research base for nursing care*. London: Scutari.

Annotated Further Reading

Wade, D. (1992) *Measurement in Neurological Rehabilitation*. Oxford: Oxford University Press.

> *This book gives a comprehensive overview of many of the available tests and scales.*

Hoeman, S. (1996) *Rehabilitation Nursing: Process and Application*, 2nd edn. St. Louis: Mosby.

> *Gives an in-depth account of rehabilitation nursing including assessment.*

O'Sullivan, S.B., & Schmitz, T.J. (eds) (1994) *Physical Rehabilitation: Assessment and Treatment*, 3rd edn, Philadelphia: F.A. Davis.

> *This book gives detailed discussion of the practice of assessment by the multi-disciplinary team and examples of assessment instruments.*

Gresham, G.E., Duncan, P.W., Stason, W.B., et al. (1993) *Post-Stroke Rehabilitation: Assessment, Referral and Patient Management*. Clinical Practice Guidelines. Quick reference guide for clinicians, no. 16. US Department of Health and Human Services, Public Health Service, Agency for Health Care Policy and Research. AHCPR number 95–0663, May 1995.

> *This includes an excellent table with references about the reliability and validity of various assessment instruments. The text is available from the Agency for Health Care Policy and Research, PO Box 8547, Silver Spring, Maryland, 20907-8547, USA or via the internet on hppt:www.tricon.net/Org/netahec/guidelines/16/*

5 Nursing diagnosis

Kaye Miller, Susan White

Key issues
- Historical perspective
- Definition and terminology
- Implementation of nursing diagnosis
- Rehabilitation nursing diagnosis
- Development opportunities and future directions

Introduction

The aim of this chapter is to discuss the definitions and terms, reasons for development, historical perspective and current status of the research and development of nursing diagnosis. Examples of the use of nursing diagnoses in clinical practice, and the opportunities for their integration within a multidisciplinary team, are given. The potential for future developments and research opportunities within the field of rehabilitation nursing are then looked at.

Historical perspective

The concept of nursing diagnosis was mentioned in nursing literature as early as 1929, when Wilson published an article in the *American Journal of Nursing* about the need to separate nursing problems from medical problems (Wilson, 1929). Even though this early date is cited in the literature, most resources on nursing diagnosis indicate that the concept began in the 1950s with the work of Fry (1953) and Abdellah (1957). They both documented the need for a system of identifying nursing problems in an organised manner. During the 1950s, nurses and paramedical professions avoided the use of diagnosis as it was seen as purely part of the medical domain. As the role of the nurse moved from the 'doctor's handmaiden' to more of an independent practitioner, nursing leaders advocated the diagnosis of nursing problems. In the USA, the term diagnosis and treatment of nursing problems was actually added to the New York State Nurse Practice Act in 1972. Many other states followed suit over the following 10 years. Another important landmark event occurred when the American Nurses Association added nursing diagnosis as a nursing function to their 1973 Standards of Nursing Practice (ANA, 1973).

Since the 1970s, the term diagnosis has no longer had only medical connotations. It is widely accepted that many different professionals will diagnose a problem from their own perspective (Miller, 1989). Progression in development of a nursing diagnosis nomenclature escalated during the 1970s, with the introduction of information technology into the health care setting. In order to include nursing contributions in computerised patient records, nurses needed to be able to classify and identify their professional practice methods, and not just provide addendum to the medical model (Miller, 1989).

In 1972, the first national conference for classifying nursing diagnosis was initiated by Gebby and Levine, and following this, Gordon became chair of a task-force on nursing diagnosis. This was instrumental in the development of nursing diagnosis in the USA until 1982, when the North American Nursing Diagnosis Association (NANDA) was created (Gordon, 1995). NANDA is an association of nursing leaders and researchers, with a special interest in nursing diagnosis. This group currently provides the administrative support for nursing diagnosis, holds bi-annual conferences and publishes revised lists of 'Approved Nursing Diagnoses' which are widely used in clinical practice throughout North America, and are being introduced into nursing education in the UK and Australia (Bennett, 1986).

Definition and terminology

Nursing diagnosis is a method of naming clients' problems which a nurse is professionally competent and registered to treat. While medical diagnosis describes the actual disease process or symptoms associated with it, the nursing diagnosis addresses the client's response to their illness or health status, which is unique for each individual client (Miller, 1989).

Each nursing diagnosis can be further differentiated into actual, risk (potential) and wellness or education diagnostic categories. NANDA has defined nursing diagnosis:

> 'A nursing diagnosis is a clinical judgment about an individual, family or community response to actual or potential health problems/life processes, which provide the basis for definitive therapy towards achievement of outcomes for which the nurse is accountable.'
>
> (Carpenito, 1991)

NANDA's format has five components; the label, definition, defining characteristics, related factors, and risk factors as detailed in Box 5.1. The format of nursing diagnosis components in Box 5.1 is very detailed and all-inclusive. This type of format is useful in developing and testing nursing diagnosis but may be difficult to follow in daily practice. Therefore, Gordon suggested a simpler format know as the PES method (Gordon, 1987). The P indicates the health problem, the E is the etiology or the related factors and the S is the signs and symptoms that guide the nurse to the selection of the problem and nursing diagnosis.

Box 5.1
*Components of a
nursing diagnosis
statement*

Label	Provides a name for a diagnosis, it is a concise term or phrase that represents a pattern of related cues. It may include qualifiers (see below).
Definition	Provides a clear, precise description, delineates its meaning, and helps differentiate it from similar diagnoses.
Defining characteristics	Observable cues and inferences that cluster as manifestation of a nursing diagnosis. These are listed for actual and wellness diagnoses. A defining characteristic is described as `critical' if it must be present to make the diagnosis and is described as `major' if it is usually present when the diagnosis exists. It is described as `minor' if it provides supporting evidence but may not be present. Critical and major defining characteristics need to be substantiated by research.
Related factors	Condition and circumstances that contribute to the development and maintenance of a nursing diagnosis.
Risk factors	Environmental factors and physiological, psychological, genetic, or chemical elements that increase the vulnerability of an individual, family or community to an unhealthful event.

(NANDA , 1994 with permission)

NANDA has classified their list of nursing diagnoses systematically, based upon their relationships to one another, in groups of nine human response patterns; exchanging, communicating, relating, valuing, choosing, moving, perceiving, knowing and feeling. The diagnosis is not a statement alone, but is a label for a related group of client problems. Functionally, the nursing diagnosis label is qualified by the related cause or contributing factors and assists the nurse in thinking through the interventions. This concept is illustrated in Case Study 5.1.

This example shows how the nursing diagnosis and 'related to' statement need to reflect the client's response to their situation, not mimic the medical diagnosis. The diagnosis label needs to stimulate clinical reasoning skills, in order that the nursing interventions can resolve the client's expressed problem. A complete list of NANDA approved nursing diagnoses is given in Appendix B.

Case study 5.1
Nursing diagnosis related to medical diagnosis

Mr Phillips has recently had a below-the-knee amputation. He has expressed his concerns about walking unsupervised on the unit, although he has been assessed for safe, independent prosthetic walking by the physiotherapist.

You have chosen the nursing diagnosis:

■ Impaired physical mobility related to left below-knee amputation.

How will you be able to plan your nursing interventions to address Mr. Phillips' problems caused by his amputation?

The problem that you have identified is related to Mr. Phillips' surgery, and will be addressed specifically by the provision of his artificial limb and ongoing physiotherapy input, rather than nursing interventions. Therefore the nursing diagnosis statement does not reflect Mr. Phillips' original concerns about walking unsupervised.

What was the primary cause of his concern? You could have selected a more appropriate nursing diagnosis of:

■ Risk of injury related to fear of falling.

Your nursing interventions would then focus on providing supervision when Mr. Phillips was walking over long distances, promoting a safe, uncluttered unit environment, and counselling about his anxieties and progress in rehabilitation treatment.

Implementation of nursing diagnosis

The implementation of a care planning system utilising the framework of nursing diagnosis is useful in clinical practice, both in providing guidance in nursing documentation and as an educational tool. Nursing diagnosis can be used in planning patient care as a part of the nursing process (Fonteyn, 1995). In 1994, the Association of Rehabilitation Nurses (ARN, 1994) published standards of care (see Box 5.2) which address the use of nursing diagnoses in care planning.

The nursing care planned and implemented for a specific nursing diagnosis is aimed at resolution or reduction of a client problem, and the nurse alone assumes responsibility and accountability for the outcome. The rehabilitation nurse identifies actual or potential nursing diagnoses from a holistic and comprehensive assessment, in consultation with the client, which addresses physical, cognitive, behavioural, emotional and developmental needs (Dean-Barr, 1993). Nursing assessment was discussed in detail in the previous chapter by Iain Bowie.

In many rehabilitation settings a multidisciplinary team approach to treatment is the most practical, because the problems are very

Box 5.2
ARN standards of care

I: Assessment	The rehabilitation nurse collects client health data.
II: Diagnosis	The rehabilitation nurse analyses the assessment data when determining diagnosis.
III: Outcome identification	The rehabilitation nurse identifies expected outcomes individualised to the client.
IV: Planning	The rehabilitation nurse develops a plan of care that prescribes interventions to attain expected outcomes.
V: Implementation	The rehabilitation nurse implements the interventions identified in the plan of care.
VI: Evaluation	The rehabilitation nurse evaluates the client's progress towards attainment of outcomes.

(Reproduced with kind permission from ARN, 1994)

complex and cannot be resolved purely by nursing interventions, but through liaison and joint treatment approaches with medical and other paramedical professions. Many rehabilitation units reflect their multidisciplinary practice through joint client records, in which nursing diagnosis has a relevant place.

The Rehabilitation Nursing Forum of the Royal College of Nursing produced Standards of Care: Rehabilitation Nursing in 1994. One of the standards is related to working within the interdisciplinary team and is as follows:

'A formal method of planning care is adopted in collaboration with the client, carers and all members of the interdisciplinary team, so that effective and realistic goal planning may be achieved.'

(RCN, 1994)

The concept of teamwork in rehabilitation settings has been previously discussed in Chapter 3 by Hilary Whitelock.

To assist the reader in fully understanding the use of this framework in care planning, two further case studies are given, the first illustrating a client with a physical problem, and the second, a cognitive or behavioural problem. These focus on a primary nursing diagnosis and are not intended to address all other nursing diagnoses for the identified clients.

Case study 5.2:
A client with an eating and swallowing problem

John Adams is a 62 year old man admitted to a stroke rehabilitation unit with a right hemisphere stroke.

From your nursing assessment, Mr. Adams is alert and orientated and although he is dysarthric he is able to communicate his basic daily needs. He has a left-sided weakness and unilateral neglect. Sitting balance is poor and he tends to lean towards the left.

Left facial weakness is noted and drooling of saliva is present. Cranial nerve assessment finds deviated tongue protrusion, an impaired gag reflex and Mr. Adams is unable to manage his own secretions effectively.

His family reports a recent weight loss.

The related nursing diagnosis to address the swallowing problems for Mr. Adams may include the following:

- Impaired swallowing
- Potential for aspiration
- Altered nutrition: less than body requirements.

Which potential nursing diagnosis is most appropriate for this client?

For Mr. Adams the nursing diagnosis most relevant in this situation is 'Potential for Aspiration'.

To complete the plan of care, select the nursing diagnosis, add a 'related to' statement, which will help to guide the interventions. At this time the nurse may wish to consult with the other appropriate team members to develop a multidisciplinary plan of care.

Nursing diagnosis: potential for aspiration related to poor swallowing reflexes and difficulty in maintaining sitting balance.

Nursing interventions will include:

- Monitor respiratory status and vital signs for early detection of infection.
- Have suction equipment readily available.
- Monitor weight and liaise with dietitian.
- Maintain nil-by-mouth and feed by nasogastric tube until swallowing assessment is complete.
- Liaise with speech language therapist for evaluation and specific oral feeding guidelines.
- Liaise with physiotherapist/occupational therapist for appropriate seating and positioning guidelines.

The Nursing interventions will be evaluated and updated as changes are identified and the client progresses. The nursing diagnosis may also change as progression is made.

If swallowing problems are resolved and the client's weight remains low, the nursing diagnosis may change to 'alteration in nutrition: less than body requirements', with the nursing interventions focusing on dietary supplementation.

This example illustrates how nursing diagnosis can assist the nurse in easy identification of the correct nursing interventions in rehabilitation care planning for stroke clients (Chipps, Clanin and Campbell, 1992; Dyker and Lees, 1996; Hickey, 1997; Kyriazis, 1994).

Case study 5.3:
A client with a behaviourally focused and sexual dysfunction problem

Ms Burns is a 27 year old female with a medical diagnosis of traumatic brain injury. She has been on the rehabilitation unit for 6 weeks. She is now alert but confused and disoriented.

Ms Burns has minimal weakness and can walk independently. She is exhibiting disinhibited behaviours, illustrated by making inappropriate sexual advances to other clients. This is causing concern and embarrassment for her family members and presents supervision problems for the staff.

Problems identified from nursing assessment include:

- Disorientation
- Confusion
- Disinhibition
- Hypersexuality
- Residual weakness.

Through the process of care planning, the potential choice of nursing diagnosis for Ms Burns could include the following categories:

- Altered sexuality patterns
- Sexual dysfunction
- Impaired cognition (Weinberg, Babicki and Miller-McIntyre, 1988. Not a NANDA approved nursing diagnosis)
- Impaired social interaction
- Acute confusion

From the assessment data, the chosen nursing diagnosis at this stage in Ms Burn's rehabilitation is 'impaired social interaction related to disinhibited behaviours secondary to traumatic brain injury'.

Nursing interventions:

- Frequently orientate to time, person, place and situation.
- Provide close supervision.
- Monitor safety.
- Liaise with neuropsychology and other members of the multidisciplinary team for management strategies for consistent redirection and orientation approach.

- ■ Family education and support.
- ■ Re-direct sexual activity to appropriate place and situation (i.e. weekend leave with significant other or privacy on unit).

In the evaluation step, if Ms Burns problems persist, the more appropriate long-term nursing diagnosis may be 'Alteration in sexuality patterns: hypersexuality related to increased libido', or 'Altered health maintenance related to choice of contraception and STD prevention'.

Rehabilitation nursing diagnosis

The Rehabilitation Nursing Foundation, in collaboration with Dr. Marjory Gordon, conducted a four-phase research study on nursing diagnosis in rehabilitation nursing practice. The results of their postal surveys of ARN members practicing in a variety of rehabilitation settings identified 21 nursing diagnoses which were common to all practitioners (see Box 5.3). The published results of this research are produced in a booklet which provides specific guidance for development of care plans in many rehabilitation settings (RNF, 1995). Other organisations have produced similar guidelines to meet the needs of their own speciality practice areas (Weinberg, Babicki and Miller-McIntyre, 1988).

Box 5.3
21 rehabilitation nursing diagnosis

1. High risk for injury
2. Impaired swallowing
3. Pressure ulcer
4. Reflex incontinence
5. Urinary retention
6. Colonic constipation
7. Feeding self-care deficit
8. Bathing or hygiene self-care deficit
9. Dressing and grooming self-care deficit
10. Toileting self-care deficit
11. Impaired physical mobility
12. Activity intolerance
13. Knowledge deficit
14. Pain
15. Impaired thought processes
16. Body image disturbance
17. Impaired verbal communication
18. Caregiver role strain
19. Ineffective individual coping
20. Ineffective family coping
21. High risk for disuse syndrome

(RNF, 1995, with permission from ARN)

The NANDA nursing diagnosis taxonomy is not a complete or exclusive list. Nurses may need to develop specific nursing diagnoses to address the problems of their own client groups. NANDA expects nurses to modify, alter and add to the currently approved list.

If a different nursing diagnosis is being used consistently in a speciality, it may be submitted to NANDA for debate and clinical review by a diagnostic review committee (DRC).

Submitted nursing diagnoses are reviewed on 4 levels: Level 1 = Received for development (consultation); Level 2 = Accepted for clinical development (authentication/substantiation); Level 3 = Clinically supported (validation and testing); Level 4 = Revision (refinement).

This review process includes studies which aim to establish the validity and clinical application of new nursing diagnoses. The inclusion of a nursing diagnosis framework for care planning may help to demonstrate that nursing practice is indeed evidence-based.

Further information on this process can be obtained from NANDA at the address given in Appendix A.

Development opportunities and future directions

At the present time, the use of a nursing diagnosis framework can be helpful in clinical practice by consolidating care planning skills. It provides a reference point for clinical reasoning, for staff new to rehabilitation, and can enhance the care-planning skills of the more experienced staff. Clinical reasoning varies from the traditional nursing process, as it facilitates the experienced nurse to analyse interrelated client problems and to plan integrated care. The nursing process method, however, focuses attention on each specific client problem, with care plans written separately with little reference to each other (Fonteyn, 1995). The use of nursing diagnosis in clinical supervision may assist the less experienced staff to apply clinical reasoning skills to the care planning process (Hickey, 1997).

Advocates of nursing diagnosis also use the framework as a basis for clinical audit, to improve consistency and content of documentation. In the USA, external accreditation organisations use the nursing diagnosis framework as a point of reference in documentation review and it is addressed in their standards guidelines (CARF, 1996; JCAHO, 1996).

The recent inception of clinical pathways as a method of recording and providing care has also changed traditional care-planning documentation. Clinical pathways are generally developed in rehabilitation for specific disability groups and have pre-set goals and interventions, over a defined time frame. A client is admitted to a rehabilitation 'pathway', with set medical and therapeutic interventions and goals that must be completed on a daily or weekly basis. The concept of clinical pathways was developed in response to purchasers' demands for a reduction in length of clients' stay and the need to standardise service provision.

A defined clinical pathway can be interrupted by unexpected complications which are referred to as variances. The use of nursing diagnosis to effectively treat and manage the variance will allow the pathway to be resumed. For example, a client on a clinical pathway for spinal cord injury may develop a pressure sore, which would increase length of stay and divert multidisciplinary care from the pathway. Nursing care aimed at treating the pressure sore in a timely and cost-effective manner will promote client recovery sufficiently to allow them to re-enter the pathway. Nursing diagnosis and pathway formats can be used together in clinical practice, as both are guides to help determine interventions and predict outcomes (Benjamin and Warner, 1996).

Conclusion

It is suggested that the future continuing use of nursing diagnosis is under debate, as the climate of health care provision continues to develop and change (Hickey, 1997). However, nursing diagnosis provides the nursing profession with a language to describe the complexities of its care and practice. From its inception, NANDA has focused on research, development and clinical testing of nursing diagnosis statements. As such, the use of nursing diagnosis in clinical practice supports the current trend towards evidence-based practice, and is easy to incorporate into the framework of clinical audit and standard setting. Therefore, the authors believe that the value of nursing diagnosis will continue to be recognised in professional practice and education.

Questions for discussion

- Having read about the development of nursing diagnosis in North America, discuss how this concept could be developed in the UK.
- A criticism of nursing diagnoses is the use of negative words such as 'impaired', 'deficit,' and 'ineffective' within the problem statement. Consider how you can promote a more positive care plan statement through goal planning.
- Identify the potential nursing diagnoses which you could introduce into the model of nursing in your practice area.
- Review the approved list of nursing diagnoses; can you identify other possible nursing diagnoses for your speciality which might be suitable for submission to NANDA?

References

Abdellah, F. (1957) Methods of identifying covert aspects of nursing problems. *Nursing Research*, **6**, 4–23.

American Nurses' Association (1973) *American Nurses' Association Standards of Practice.* Kansas MI: American Nurses' Association.

Association of Rehabilitation Nurses (ARN) (1994) *Standards and Scope of Rehabilitation Nursing*

Practice, 3rd edn. Stokie IL: Association of Rehabilitation Nurses. With permission of the Association of Rehabilitation Nurses, 4700 W. Lake Avenue, Glenview, IL 60025–1485. Copyright © 1994.

Benjamin, J. & Warner, B. (1996) Principles of leadership and management. In *Rehabilitation Nursing: Process and Application*, ed. Hoeman, S., pp. 70–86. St. Louis: Mosby.

Bennett, M. (1986) Nursing Diagnosis: in the beginning. *Australian Journal of Advanced Nursing*, **4**, 41–46.

Commission of Accreditation of Rehabilitation Facilities (1996) *Standards for Accreditation*. Phoenix AZ: (CARF).

Carpenito, L. (1991) The NANDA definition of nursing diagnosis. In *Classification of Nursing Diagnoses; Proceedings of the Ninth Conference*, ed. Carroll-Johnson, R. M. Philadelphia: J. B. Lippincott.

Chipps, E., Clanin, N. & Campbell, V. (1992) *Neurological Disorders*. St. Louis: Mosby.

Dean-Baar, S. (1993) Application of the new ANA framework for nursing practice standards and guidelines. *Journal of Nursing Care Quality*, **8**, 33–42.

Dyker, A. & Lees, K. (1996) Advances in therapy for stroke. *Hospital Update*, **22**, 287–293.

Fonteyn, M. (1995) Clinical reasoning in nursing. In *Clinical Reasoning in Health Professions*, eds. Higgs, J. & Jones, M. pp. 60–71. Oxford: Butterworth-Heinemann.

Fry, V. S. (1953) The creative approach to nursing. *American Journal of Nursing*, **53**, 301–302.

Gordon, M. (1995) *Manual of Nursing Diagnosis*. St. Louis: Mosby.

Gordon, M. (1987) *Nursing Diagnosis: Process and Application*, 2nd edn. New York: McGraw-Hill.

Hickey, J. (1997) *The Clinical Practice of Neurological and Neurosurgical Nursing*, 4th edn. Philadelphia: Lippincott-Raven.

Joint Commission on the Accreditation of Hospitals (JCOAH) (1996) *Accreditation Manual for Hospitals*. Chicago, IL: JCOAH.

Kyriazis, M. (1994) Developments in the treatment of stroke patients. *Nursing Times*, **90**, 30–31.

Miller, E. (1989) *How to Make Nursing Diagnosis Work*. Norwalk, CT: Appleton & Lange.

North American Nursing Diagnosis Association (1994) *Guidelines for Nursing Diagnosis Submission*. Philadelphia: North American Nursing Diagnosis Association.

Royal College of Nursing (1994) *Standards of Care: Rehabilitation Nursing*, London: RCN.

Rehabilitation Nursing Foundation (1995). *21 Rehabilitation Nursing Diagnoses: A Guide to Interventions and Outcomes*. With permission of the Association of Rehabilitation Nurses, 4700 W. Lake Avenue, Glenview, IL 60025–1485. Copyright © 1995. Illinois: Rehabilitation Nursing Foundation.

Weinberg, L., Babicki, C. & Miller-McIntrye, K. (1988) *Rehabilitation Nursing Care Plan Stimulators*. Washington, DC: National Rehabilitation Hospital.

Wilson, F. (1929) Nursing medical patients: an analysis of problems encountered by student nurses in caring for them. *American Journal of Nursing*, **29**, 245.

Annotated further reading

Chipps, E., Clanin, N. & Campbell V. (1992) *Neurological Disorders*, pp. 738–781. St. Louis: Mosby.

D'Argenio, C. (1991) *Implementing Nursing Diagnosis Based Practice*. Maryland: Aspen Publishers Inc.

Dyker, A. & Lees, K. (1996) Advances in therapy for stroke. *Hospital Update*, **22**, 287–293.

Hickey, J. (1997) *The Clinical Practice of Neurological and Neurosurgical Nursing*, 4th edn. Philadelphia: Lippincott-Raven.

Hoeman, S. (1996) *Rehabilitation Nursing: Process and Application, 2nd edn*, pp. 354–360. St. Louis: Mosby.

Kyriazis, M. (1994) Developments in the treatment of stroke patients. *Nursing Times*, **90**, 30–31.

   Texts to assist in nursing diagnosis in planning care for clients after stroke.

Grindell, P., Le Blanc, L. & Cawley, D. (1996) Operationalizing a comprehensive neurobehavioural plan. *Rehabilitation Nursing*, **21**, 91–93, 97.

Helgadottir, H. L. (1996) Psychosocial issues following serious head injury: a case study of an adolescent girl. *Rehabilitation Nursing*, **21**, 258–261.

Stratton, M. C. & Gregory, R. J. (1995) What happens after a traumatic brain injury: four case studies. *Rehabilitation Nursing*, **20**, 323–327.

   Further reading for using nursing diagnosis in the management of clients following brain injury.

6 Setting goals in rehabilitation

Sally Davis

Introduction

Within rehabilitation, the setting of interdisciplinary goals is becoming recognised as a method which promotes client empowerment and ensures maximum effectiveness of the rehabilitation process. Although an aspect of the nurse's role in any health care setting is concerned with the setting of goals when planning care for clients, it is difficult to discuss goal setting in rehabilitation nursing without setting it in the context of the interdisciplinary team. This chapter will examine the concept of goal setting and the issues surrounding the planning and implementation of goals for clients, relatives, and professionals. Implications for nurses will continually be addressed throughout the chapter.

What is goal setting?

Goal setting is not a new concept, it is something that we all do in every-day life in order to achieve our aims. Locke (1968) identifies goal directedness as being a distinctive feature of rational human activity. Goal setting has been seen as a key concept in the field of organisational management for some time. Business planning is a good example where goals are set for the forthcoming year, taking into account the resources available. In health care, business planning is one aspect of management that is having to be taken on board, not only by managers but by the clinical team.

Theories and models

Edwin Locke (1968) formulated a goal setting theory which assumes that motivation is a result of rational and intentional behaviour. Goals can direct attention, mobilise effort, increase persistence and motivate strategy development, all of which can affect performance (Locke et al., 1981). Maslow's (1968), hierarchy of needs, based on the same premises as Locke's theory, describes a person as being motivated to direct behaviour toward meeting each successive layer of individual needs, as identified in his hierarchy. Maslow's hierarchy is fairly well known by nurses and is often used in the setting of nursing/client goals. It can be used to help assess a client's priorities and motivation.

McGrath and Davis (1992) classify models related to goal setting under two main types: the machine model of human problem solving, which is within the field of experimental psychology (Newell and Simon, 1963) and effective action models, which are within the field of organisational management (McGregor, 1960). McGrath and Davis (1992) identify both of these types of models as involving five stages:

- selecting the goal
- analysing the task
- making decisions
- initiating action
- evaluating the previous four stages.

Each stage is dependent on the previous one and the results of evaluation are fed back to the earlier stages. These five stages can give professionals a structure on which to set goals with clients.

Theory of goal attainment

Imogene King (1981), a nursing theorist, identified a conceptual framework or model which viewed personal, interpersonal and social systems. The focus of King's model is on the attainment of goals through interaction. King (1981) defines nursing as being:

> *'A process of human interactions between nurse and client whereby each perceives the other and the situation; and through communication, they set goals, explore means, and agree on means to achieve goals.'*

> (King, 1981 p. 144).

The goal of nursing is identified as being to help individuals function in their roles by assisting them in maintaining their health (King, 1981). King makes some assumptions about nurse–client interactions, which are listed in Box 6.1.

Box 6.1
Dynamics of nurse – client interactions

- The interaction process is influenced by the values, needs, goals and perceptions of the nurse and client.
- Clients have a right to participate in decisions that influence their life and they also have a right to knowledge about themselves.
- Health professionals have a responsibility to share information with clients to enable them to make informed decisions about their health care.
- Goals of clients and health care professionals may not be congruent.

Within this model there is a strong interactive basis with a goal-setting emphasis, which is appropriate for rehabilitation nurses. Although aimed at nurses, the goal of nursing action, which is to interact purposefully with clients to mutually establish goals and the means for achieving them, could be identified as being the goal for the whole team.

The nursing process

Goal setting is included in the nursing process and provides nurses with a rational way of organising information so that care given is appropriate and effective (Leddy and Pepper, 1989). The nursing process is a systematic, problem-solving process of assessment, planning and evaluation. It is the goals or objectives identified from the nursing diagnosis (see Chapter 6) which determine the nursing outcomes that are expected as a result of implementation of the planned care (Leddy and Pepper, 1989).

Conceptual nursing models are systematically constructed, scientifically based, logically related sets of concepts which identify the essential components of nursing practice (Leddy and Pepper, 1989). They provide nurses with a knowledge base which should be congruent with their own beliefs and values about their client group. The nursing process remains unchanged regardless of which nursing model nurses choose. However, the aims of goal setting may be different in each model, as identified by Leddy and Pepper (1989) (see Table 6.1).

It could be said that all of these guidelines are conducive with the aim of rehabilitation. However, goal setting within Roper's model of activities of daily living (Roper 1976), which many nurses in the UK use to guide their practice, can be identified as being limiting with its focus on the acquirement and restoration of independence in activities of daily living.

Table 6.1
Nursing models: guidelines for goal setting (adapted from Leddy and Pepper, 1989)

Nursing model	Broad guidelines for goal setting
Orem	Restore internal and external consistency
Roy	Promote adaptation from successful coping
Neuman	Maintain or restore the dynamic equilibrium of the normal line of defense
King	Achieve personal, interpersonal and social goals

Relationship of goal setting to rehabilitation

Rehabilitation can be identified as being a reiterative problem-solving educational process which focuses on disability and aims to reduce handicap and client and family distress, while keeping within the limitations imposed by the pathology and resources available (Wade, 1996). This definition is based on the World Health

Organisation's (1980) classification of impairments, disabilities and handicaps (ICIDH).

The processes involved within rehabilitation are assessment, planning, intervention and reassessment. Wade (1996) identifies the area of planning as causing professionals the most difficulty. It is not easy to set realistic goals which are meaningful to the client and will enable them to achieve a quality of life which is acceptable to them. In the past, the setting of goals has tended to be on a more ad-hoc basis, dictated by professionals. This is normally a characteristic of a multidisciplinary team approach where professionals are focusing more on the level of disability, which does not allow for much overlapping of roles. This has resulted in disjointed goals which have not been aimed at the level of handicap.

Interdisciplinary goal setting can enable a team to achieve the elements of an effective team, as identified by Embling (1995), by enabling shared goals, interdependence, overlap of roles, cooperation between all members of the team, coordination of activities, division of effort, mutual respect and task specialisation. This, in turn, then enables clients and families to feel that the rehabilitation programme is aimed at goals they themselves want to achieve. The aim is for them to feel that they are at the centre of the rehabilitation process.

Advantages of goal setting

Empowerment

The concept of empowerment is often identified by nurses as being a nursing goal. It is a complex concept with many implications that are often paid lip-service to. Goal setting can be seen as being a way to give control back to clients and make empowerment real. If rehabilitation is to be about helping individuals achieve a quality of life and to return to former or new roles, then there has to be a move away from a medical approach to one that focuses on health promotion, where the emphasis is on wellness rather than illness, and which seeks to empower individuals (Naidoo and Wills, 1994). This move has to be made by all nurses and other professionals within the team.

Rodwell (1996) identifies empowerment as being a process which enables groups or individuals to change after being given the skills, resources, opportunities and authority to do so. It is a partnership where there is a transferring of power, which enables the development of a positive self esteem and the recognition of worth of self and others. Clients going through the rehabilitation process often feel worthless and have low self esteem. They go through a long phase of adaptation and for some, this phase is never reconciled. Empowerment can be a way of giving them back some power and thereby some self esteem. Goal setting can enable clients and professionals to feel motivated. Individuals in general feel satisfaction when they have worked towards and achieved a goal.

The defining attributes of empowerment, as identified by Rodwell (1996), are:

- It is a helping process
- It is a partnership which values self and others
- It involves mutual decision-making using resources, opportunities and authority:
- It confers freedom to make choices and accept responsibility.

In a visual representation of an empowerment model for nursing. Gibson (1991) identifies client – nurse interactions as being ones of: trust, empathy, participatory decision-making, mutual goal setting, cooperation, negotiation, overcoming organisational barriers, lobbying and legitimacy. They identify the nurse as being a helper, counselor, educator, resource consultant, facilitator, enabler, advocate, and a giver of support.

These interactions and domains can assist nurses and other professionals in identifying what kind of interactions and roles are conducive to an empowering approach. Because of nurses' 24-hour responsibility for clients, it is essential that all of the nursing team are consistent in using an empowering approach.

Focus on client's goals

Goal setting enables goals to be focused on the client rather than on the professional, and can enable the client, carers and the team to focus on the client's strengths rather than their problems. The team can guide the client into thinking of goals at the level of handicap, rather than disability and therefore take a more long-term view. It is important that nursing-specific goals address not only the level of disability but also the level of handicap, so that they are in line with the philosophy behind goal setting. For example, they have to take into account an individual's expectations for the future, their potential quality of life at home, social activities, etc.

Client-centred goals enable the team to identify where the client and their family are in their thinking regarding their rehabilitation programme, and whether they are focusing on realistic goals or not. The team are then in a better position to help clients and their relatives adapt to their situation and reinforce or alter goals and aims.

Task performance

Literature shows that task performance is affected by goal setting. Locke et al. (1981) summarised research relating the effects of setting various types of goals on task performance. They found that 90% of the studies they examined showed positive or partial positive effects of goal setting on task performance, as long as the goals were specific and sufficiently challenging. McGrath and Davis (1992) emphasise that the stages of goal selection and task analysis are not completely independent. The language in which goals are stated may determine the form task analysis takes, and it is important that goals are stated clearly to avoid duplication of activity.

Interdisciplinary team

As mentioned previously, goal setting enables the team to work in more of an interdisciplinary way, where the focus is on the level of handicap and there is overlap of roles (McGrath and Davis, 1992). It enables collaboration to take place by the formulation of common objectives to problem-solve between the professionals, the client and their family, which in itself encourages interdisciplinary team working and client empowerment. Interdisciplinary team working is covered in more depth in Chapter 3.

Goal setting forces professionals to explore how they communicate with each other. The process will be ineffective if communication is poor. It is important that nurses work together as a team and that they are clear as to what their role is within the interdisciplinary team. It is also important that other members of the team understand their role. Issues of role conflict and role overlap will need to be constructively explored and strategies identified to minimise these.

The process of goal setting

There are a number of issues that need to be considered carefully when implementing the goal setting process:

- vocabulary used
- involvement of the client and their family
- roles of the team within the goal setting process
- goal setting meeting
- incompatibility of goals
- staff training
- evaluation of the process.

Vocabulary

In order for goal setting to be effective, it is important that all of the team have the same understanding of the meanings of the terms used within the process. Davis et al. (1992) identified a general lack of consensus in the literature regarding the definition of goals, which were referred to as desires, purposes, ambitions, wishes, aims, needs, steps, plans, values, proximal and distal goals, expectations and short- and long-term goals. Locke (1969) identifies the following concepts which have similar meanings to that of 'goal':

- performance standard: a measuring rod for evaluating performance
- quota: a minimum amount of work or production
- work norm: a standard of acceptable behaviour defined by a work group
- task: a piece of work to be accomplished
- objective: the ultimate aim of an action or series of actions

- deadline: a time limit for completing a task
- budget: a spending goal or limit.

Elements from all of the above concepts can be interpreted to be useful for goal setting within rehabilitation.

Performance standard
The setting of goals can be identified as being a means of measuring the client's performance in meeting identified goals and the professional's performance in enabling clients to meet these goals.

Quota
This could be identified as being related to the work norm which would need to include a minimum amount of work which could be expected by the team for each client. For example, this could be a stated amount of therapy input, or related to the facilitation of a rehabilitating environment, or certain minimum requirements that can be expected by all clients regardless of their own objectives.

Work norm
In order for the team to work in an interdisciplinary way, they need to identify what their standard of acceptable behaviour needs to be in order to meet their service requirements. Strategies such as a team philosophy and a mission statement for the unit will help them identify these standards.

Task
The task will be the work that needs to be accomplished in order for clients to achieve their goals, and may be referred to as targets. McGrath and Marks (1995) identify a target as being:

> 'A measurable, observable state or action set in a short time-frame, which is a necessary step towards the achievement of objectives'.

Objective
A number of small tasks may need to be achieved in order to meet the objective of the client's rehabilitation programme, which will be the ultimate aim. McGrath and Marks (1995) identify an objective as being a:

> 'Change which can be achieved within a specified time-frame. It may be a role behaviour, or may relate to changing the expectations of the client or carers. It is a necessary step towards the achievement of an aim'.

Deadline
It is important to identify a realistic time limit for each identified task. If the task has not been achieved within the time limit it is important for the team to evaluate why.

Budget
It could be destructive if clients identify objectives which are agreed by the team, even though the team knows they do not have the resources either in staff time or budget to meet them.

McGrath and Marks (1995), in their definition of terms, also identify the term aim as being:

'An expected, or hoped-for, state which encompasses a role or roles and the environment, which can be reached within a reasonable time. Aims should refer to the areas considered most important by the client, and incorporate maximum freedom of choice within these areas'.

Davis et al. (1992) identify aims as being described in terms of handicap and social role, with objectives being the steps to achieve the aims. Objectives are then broken down into targets. Objectives are interdisciplinary, being achieved by more than one member of the team, with targets being the steps each professional needs to take to achieve the objectives. Therefore, specific nursing objectives needed to achieve the interdisciplinary objective would be seen as targets.

An example of an aim could be:

'For Ann to return to live at home with her family independently.'

For which one objective would be:

'For Ann to be independent in preparing snacks.'

The objective would be one of many to achieve the aim. In the objective chosen, a number of professionals may be involved in helping Ann achieve it, e.g. occupational therapist, physiotherapist, nurse. Each professional will then identify targets to meet the objective. For example a nursing target might be:

'For Ann to get her own breakfast each morning on the ward.'

Nursing action would then need to be identified to achieve this target. Objectives, goals and targets are recognised terms within the field of management, often being referred to in terms of SMART (specified, motivating, attainable, rational, timed) and RUMBA (relevant, understandable, measurable, behavioural, attainable). Schut and Stam (1994) summarise these criteria resulting in requirements for goal setting. Goals should be:

- relevant, motivating, positively defined and should express what is wanted to be accomplished
- Explicit and commonly understandable, expressed in behavioural terms
- Attainable and enable well-balanced planning and measurement.

Relating the setting of goals to the rehabilitation setting, applying the above requirements, will result in goals being expressed as activities that are of value for the client and that can be achieved in a planned time span. Attention needs to be paid to the differences between the value of activities for the client and the professional (Schut and Stam, 1994).

Involvement of client and family

The most important element of the goal setting process is the involvement of the client and their family. As already stated, goal setting in itself is a way of empowering clients. Promoting client involvement in health care is not a new concept. The nursing process and certain models of nursing have promoted the involvement of clients in their care to give them more control (Smith and Draper, 1994). Client involvement has also been the focus of individual and clients' rights movements (Tyne, 1994). There has been a shift in thinking in rehabilitation settings in the UK to involving clients in their care rather than telling them what to do. This equates with a wellness model approach to health care, where the focus is on enabling clients to be empowered (Armentrout, 1993), rather than an illness model approach.

Malin & Teasdale (1991) conducted a qualitative study which focused on the tensions between the concepts of caring and empowerment. In this study, caring is identified as having the related concepts of altruism, control and paternalism which are at odds with the idea of empowerment, which places the client in a partnership relationship. Although this study was directed at nurses, these notions could apply to any health care professional in a caring role.

For clients to be involved in the rehabilitation process, a shift in thinking needs to take place in the members of the team, with them identifying their role as being something other than caring. Enabling would seem to be a concept more in line with empowerment and intimates that professionals will use strategies which will enable clients to be empowered and begin to take control over what is happening to them. This change of emphasis from doing to enabling can be particularly difficult for nurses to achieve, as nursing is commonly thought of as caring, with nurses in more of a 'doing for' role. Even though this notion may be changing within the nursing profession, it is often still the perception of the media, clients and relatives.

Members of the team need to establish a relationship with the client and their family where there is mutual respect. Research has shown that greater levels of goal attainment are achieved when mutual goal setting takes place (Galano, 1977; Ventura et al., 1983; Willer and Miller, 1976). Historically, nurses have always been warned against becoming too involved with clients. However, it is not possible to have a relationship where there is mutual goal setting when it is only the client who is giving something of themselves.

Team members need to develop an inner awareness of their own values that may influence the setting of goals for individual clients (Urbanowski and Vargo, 1994). Conversely, it is important that the team are aware of any values and beliefs that the client and their family may hold which will have a bearing on the goal setting process. Urbanowski & Vargo (1994), in an article exploring the concept of spirituality for occupational therapy practice, make the point that in order to stop programmes becoming tedious regimes for the client, goals must be value-orientated rather than process-orientated, in order for them to have a true-life meaning for the client.

Solution focused brief therapy, based on psychotherapy, is an approach that identifies and works towards clients' goals, identifying the client's own strengths and resources. It is carried out in such a way to facilitate cooperation rather than conflict. This can lead to the client's own discovery of the resources they have which they can use to deal with the problems they are experiencing (Iveson, 1994).

The principles of solution focused brief therapy (Iveson, 1994) can be used as a guide for discussion with the client in a rehabilitation setting:

Description of the task

The professional needs to describe what their task is in a language the client can understand. For example, their task could be to enable the client to identify goals which are meaningful to them. This then needs to be put into the client's perspective, e.g. relating it to their life and the events that have happened to them.

An interest in the client's past

In order to have an understanding of the client as an individual person, of their beliefs, values and coping strategies, knowing what the client has achieved in their life and what difficult times they have coped with, will give the team an insight into their strengths, their coping strategies and their inner resources.

An interest in the client's future

It may be necessary to help the client adjust their aspirations for the future in light of their new circumstances.

What should the client's involvement be? Is it realistic for them to set their own goals? Jelles, van Bennekom and Lankhorst (1995) argue that this is not tenable, as clients who have been confronted with disease or injury cannot be expected to judge their situation validly. Clients are often depressed, disorientated, demoralised and anxious in the first stages of rehabilitation (Caplan, 1988; Hass, 1993). It is often not possible in the early stages for them to know what the consequences for them will be, which will result in uncertainties for them and their relatives (Caplan, 1988; Haas, 1993). The educational model (van Bennekom, Jelles and Lankhorst, 1995) focuses on professionals teaching the client to make their own decisions and be responsible for those decisions. This approach is synonymous with the following principles of adult learning as identified by Ingram (1981 cited in Ventura et al. 1984).

- Adults need a clear understanding of the goal they are working towards and the means to achieve it.
- Adults need feedback on the progress they have made towards the goal.

■ Adults need to feel that they are progressing in order to feel motivated.

■ If given a set of criteria, adults can evaluate their own performance.

The educational model is similar to the health promotion model of education, where the aim is to provide knowledge and information and to develop the necessary skills so that the client can make an informed choice (Naidoo and Wills, 1994). This is contrary to the medical or paternalistic model (van Bennekom, et al., 1995) where the professionals are responsible for the rehabilitation process with goals being set without client involvement.

If client's needs are to be taken into account then it is important that professionals identify any constraints that there may be to the client being involved in goal setting, and that a plan is formulated to address how involvement will be achieved. They need to assess the client's readiness to receive information and learn new skills. It may be necessary for the professionals to have greater control at the beginning of the process, with the emphasis changing to give more control to the client. This is supported by Price (1986), who identifies the shift in control for clients as they go through the process of rehabilitation, with the team having the major control at the beginning of the rehabilitation process but with this slowly changing to the client having the most control.

In an attempt to involve clients at the beginning of the process of rehabilitation at the Rivermead Rehabilitation Centre (RRC) in Oxford, a life goals questionnaire was devised (Figure 6.1) which is loosely based on a life satisfaction questionnaire by Fugl-Meyer, Branholm and Fugl-Meyer, (1991). The questionnaire enables staff to focus on what the client identifies as being the most important aspects of their life (Davis et al. 1992).

Roles of the team

The issues surrounding the team are explored in detail in Chapter 3. However, it is important to consider the roles of the team within the goal setting process. In order for the team to function in an interdisciplinary way, they need to have a common understanding of each other's roles. The roles of individual team members and the issues around role conflict are also discussed in Chapter 3. The team need to have common beliefs and values about the process of goal planning, e.g. if one member of the team does not believe in empowerment for clients and is operating in more of a medical model framework where they are taking control, then this will be destructive for the whole process. Strategies such as a unit philosophy, job descriptions that reflect the philosophy and an overall goal or mission statement for the unit can help minimise this potential problem.

Figure 6.1
Life goals question-naire from the Rivermead Rehabilitation Centre, Oxford, 1998 (with permission from Rivermead Rehabilitation Centre)

Various aspects and areas of life are given below. I would like you to tell me how important each is to you. Please rate the importance of each: 0 = of no importance Date completed:_____ 1 = of some importance 2 = of great importance Interviewer:_____ 3 = of extreme importance Comments		
My residential and domestic arrangements (where I live and who with) are:	0 1 2 3	
My ability to manage my personal care (dressing, toilet, washing) is:	0 1 2 3	
My leisure, hobbies and interests including pets are:	0 1 2 3	
My work, paid or unpaid is:	0 1 2 3	
My relationship with my partner (or my wish to have one) is:	0 1 2 3	
My family life (including with those not living at home) is:	0 1 2 3	
My contacts with friends, neighbours and acquaintances are:	0 1 2 3	
My religion or life philosophy is:	0 1 2 3	
My financial status is:	0 1 2 3	

As well as having their own professional role, team members will need to take on other roles, for example those of negotiator, collaborator, educator, roles that are identified within the framework of health promotion and roles that are central for client involvement. As well as these roles, team members may need to take on transient roles such as coordinator or chairperson for goal setting meetings. It is necessary to consider where the role of primary nurse and key-worker fit into the goal setting process.

Primary nurse   The crux of the primary nurse role is their responsibility for their named clients (Manthey, 1980) giving them the opportunity to develop a unique, holistic relationship with the client and their family. The role of the primary nurse in rehabilitation should be one of enabling and education, regardless of whether goal setting is in place. Within goal setting, the role of the primary nurse could be maximised to take more of a pivotal role. For example, at the RRC it is normally the primary nurses who instigate the process of goal setting, by enabling clients to complete the life goals questionnaire. It is a skillful role in enabling the client to identify those roles that are meaningful to them, without influencing them. It can be particularly difficult not to influence a client with communication or cognitive difficulties. It might be appropriate for another member of the team in this instance to facilitate the questionnaire, for example, the speech therapist or psychologist. Or if a client is particularly depressed, the psychiatrist might be the appropriate choice.

Key worker

The role of the keyworker within the goal setting process is to be responsible for a client throughout their stay, coordinating goal plans and ensuring that they are carried out (Golding and Allen, 1990). The keyworker needs to have a good working relationship with their allocated client, but also needs to keep an objective view, to ensure that they are also keeping the needs of the service in mind. One of the difficulties when working as an interdisciplinary team is the area of role conflict and of differing values and beliefs. There could also be difficulty with professionals becoming too involved in their client's programme. It is imperative that there is consistency within the team so that all clients are treated fairly within the resources available. The advantage of a keyworker is that they would be responsible for ensuring that goals are met, that they are client centred and that discharge planning is effective. It could be seen as being more effective in having one person to take on this responsibility for each patient. Where primary nursing is in place there could be seen to be overlap of roles, or the primary nurse could be identified as being the keyworker.

Dawson and Bartlett (1996) describe the introduction of a keyworker role into a Regional Neurological Unit to improve communication with regards to the discharge process. Protocol was developed which gave the keyworker power to impose deadlines on key members concerned with the production of the report and also the opportunity to facilitate interdisciplinary communication via a planning meeting. At the East Finchley Neuro-rehabilitation Unit in London, the keyworker role has been in system for the last 4 years

Box 6.2
The keyworker role at East Finchley Neuro-rehabilitation Unit

The keyworker model is not discipline specific and fulfills many purposes. It is recognised as a high-profile role with an associated degree of accountability, contributing to empowering the client/family, facilitating consensus, coordinating the team's efforts, ensuring audit standards are met, and in some cases, having an educational and unit management component. Staff from all disciplines and at all levels are eligible to act as keyworkers after appropriate in-service training and development in the role and when, in the case of junior staff, their manager feels they have the appropriate skills. Each staff member keyworks one, or at most two clients at any time, attending all the multidisciplinary team meetings, liaising with the client, helping to reinforce the aims of their rehabilitation and taking overall responsibility for facilitating consensus between team members and with the client.

They coordinate the team's efforts in discharge planning, ensuring joint reports to community teams and referers are completed in good time and despatched according to unit standards. In addition, they contribute to and oversee the team's completion of the Integrated Care Pathway (ICP) audit documentation, acting as a contact point for carers/external agencies and having an up-to-date overview of the situation at all times. Responsibility for making client referrals remains with treating team members and no keyworker makes decisions without prior discussion with the team.

The generic model, whereby a speech therapist can carry out the role as well as a nurse, a physiotherapist, occupational therapist, psychologist, doctor or social worker, was chosen as a leveler of professions within the team. This also means that extra burdens of coordination, communication and chasing administrative detail are shared, and do not fall solely to the nursing team. In addition, it can be a useful management tool, enabling senior team members, including clinical managers, to keep in touch with all aspects of the rehabilitation process experienced by individual clients. By continuous liaison with the client/family and attendance at all working team meetings, senior keyworkers can identify areas within the system for further development and potential issues for in-service training. Skilled senior clinicians also act as role models and by regularly working alongside junior staff of all disciplines, they are able to further reinforce the unit's philosophy of care.

(Jane Johnson, Clinical Nurse Specialist, Neuro-rehabilitation)

The goal setting meeting

in the format described in Box 6.2.

It is important to consider how and where goals will be set. The relationship between goal setting and an interdisciplinary approach has already been discussed as has the importance of the process involving the relevant members of the team, the client and their family. There needs to be an identified format which would enable this collaboration to take place, for example a goal setting meeting. The purpose of such a meeting can be identified as being to give the team the opportunity to share information, to collaborate and to negotiate goals with the client and their family.

The vocabulary as already discussed needs to be understood by all of the professionals involved. Everyone needs to attach the same meaning to the terms, otherwise the meeting will become ineffective.

All of the professionals need to be prepared for the meeting, coming with an idea of what the client wants to achieve and a realistic time scale. Thought needs to be given to potential discrepancies in the goals of the client, family and members of the team.

Involvement of the client and their family in the meeting needs to be considered. Should they be involved in every goal setting meeting? Should they be involved from the beginning of the meeting? It seems to go against the philosophy behind goal setting if the client and their family are not involved in the meeting. However, maybe this needs to be considered against resources available. For example, the involvement of the client and family in the meeting could increase the amount of time it will take. It may also be inappropriate to involve them in the first goal setting meeting when they may not be ready to discuss and negotiate goals with a number of people.

Who will chair the meeting? Is it appropriate that it is the consultant in an interdisciplinary team? Could it be rotated? Will all staff have the skills to chair such a meeting? How will the meeting be documented and where will these notes be kept?

Rivermead Rehabilitation Centre (RRC) in Oxford began to implement the change from a multidisciplinary to an interdisciplinary approach in the early 1990s, which included the development of interdisciplinary goal setting (McGrath and Davis, 1992; Davis et al. 1992; McGrath and Marks, 1995). Box 6.3 gives a description of how

Box 6.3
Rivermead Rehabilitation Centre's goal setting meetings

> The goal setting meeting takes place 2–3 weeks following the client's admission to the unit. A date for the meeting is negotiated at the weekly ward round and is organised at a time when all of the professionals concerned can attend. Before the meeting, the primary nurses will have interviewed the client and completed the life goals questionnaire. Combined with the questionnaire are questions which ask the client to consider their strengths and their expectations of Rivermead. The social worker or primary nurse also interviews the family asking them specific questions. All of the professionals will come to the meeting with an idea of what the client wants to achieve and what is realistically achievable. It will have been decided at ward round whether it is appropriate for the client and their family to be involved in the meeting itself. Generally they are not involved in the first meeting but are in subsequent meetings.
>
> At the meeting, someone will be appointed chairperson. It is their job to lead the meeting, to identify objectives from previous meetings and to identify who will give feedback to the client and their relatives if they are not at the meeting. At the meeting, the

nurse presents the information from the life goals questionnaire and then relevant information is presented by each member of the team. This will include the client's performance in each therapy area, including the ward. Aims are set, based on the life areas identified by the client. The team sets objectives for each aim (which usually involve more than one member of the team), identifying what needs to be done, who will do it and the time it will take. Targets may be set which are usually profession-specific.

The chairperson in negotiation with the team identifies who will give feedback to the client and their family. It is the responsibility of the chairperson to record the aims, objectives and targets identified onto a special goal setting sheet. They then photocopy the sheet and distribute a copy to everyone at the meeting, including the client and their family. The original sheet goes into the client's interdisciplinary case notes.

The client and their family are interviewed before each goal setting meeting and a new life-goals questionnaire is completed. The aims and objectives are reviewed at each meeting.

Incompatibility of goals

the goal setting meeting is organised at the RRC.

Problems with goal selection may arise when there is incompatibility of goals between the client, their family and the professionals. A difference in goals between the client and the professionals may occur at any time within the process at the level of aim, objective or target. Negotiation and collaboration are vital to the goal setting process, which involves the clients' and the professionals' goals mutually moving closer together (McGrath and Davis, 1992). Breaking longer-term goals down into short-term goals can help clients realise that they have to achieve a series of steps before they achieve their ultimate goal. Often clients will then realise themselves that they are not going to achieve their original goal. This usually also applies to relatives where their expectations are unrealistic.

Between the disciplines, there needs to be consistent and agreed rationale for prioritising goals to enable the team to come to an agreement. It is important that the team are able to communicate with each other openly and frankly (McGrath and Davis, 1992). Having a team philosophy, unit objectives and being clear as to what the aim of the service is, will also help in reducing potential incompatibility of goals.

Staff training

Interdisciplinary goal setting involving the client and their family is a complex process, and in order for it to be effective, it is important that staff are prepared adequately. Staff need to know the philosophy behind goal setting and how it fits into their unit's philosophy. The language of goal setting needs to be discussed in terms understood by all of the team. Team members will need to be prepared to take an active part in the goal setting meeting and possibly take on the role of chairperson. This calls for interpersonal and management skills such as assertiveness, negotiation and collaboration. A number of skills-teaching methods can be used to train staff to take part in goal setting, e.g. videos, workshops, group discussions and practical exercises (Golding and Allen, 1990). It is important that training is not just a one-off but is an ongoing programme giving staff the opportunity to discuss any difficulties that may arise.

Evaluation of the goal setting process

If goal setting is to be an effective, dynamic process, it is important that continuous evaluation of the process takes place. Evaluation needs to be an integral part of the system to enable modification of practice to take place in response to changes in circumstances and the level of effectiveness of the given intervention (McGrath and Davis, 1992). It is important that the evaluation includes those areas of the process which are likely to cause problems (McGrath and Marks 1995), for example:

- user friendliness of the process for staff and clients, including the terms used
- setting aims in terms of handicap
- the involvement of more than one discipline in the achievement of objectives and in the planning of therapy sessions
- recording of the wishes of the client in an accurate and meaningful way
- the relationship between the rehabilitation goals and the wishes of the client
- taking on the role of chair in the review meeting.

Evaluation of the process will assist in identifying the training needs required by the team. At the Royal National Orthopaedic Hospital in Stanmore, the goal setting process is planned as described

Box 6.4
Goal planning at the Royal National Orthopaedic Hospital, Stanmore

Goal planning is set within the framework of the unit which includes a mission statement, the meaning of rehabilitation for the unit and a unit philosophy. Each client is allocated a case manager on admission who is a member of the community liaison team. Their role is to manage and coordinate the acute, rehabilitation and reintegration process from admission to 2 years post-discharge. The case manager is responsible for:

- introducing the client to the rehabilitation process,
- explaining the process of goal planning and the eleven areas of need,
- organising and chairing all goal planning meetings and case conferences,

- acting as a focus between the client and the team, and
- record keeping and administration.

The process of rehabilitation is broken down into:

Needs   which refer to the many issues raised in daily life: physical wellbeing, accommodation, mobility, psychological wellbeing; finance, functional independence, sexuality, social reintegration, family support, self-care and independence; communication.

Goals   which refer to what the client will be doing when the needs are met.

Targets   which are the goals broken down to a finer level indicating who will do what under what conditions and to what degree of success.

The first goal planning meeting is held within 2 weeks following the client's beginning to mobilise or within 4 weeks for clients on long-term bedrest. The client, case manager, nurse, physiotherapist and occupational therapist attend the goal planning meetings which are held every 2 weeks. FIM (functional independence measure) scores are completed at the beginning of each alternate meeting. At each meeting, goals are set within the 11 areas of need which are objective, measurable and achievable. Targets are set, related to the goals. The discharge checklist is completed as appropriate and further goal planning meetings are arranged.

Case conferences are held at the beginning of the client's rehabilitation programme and prior to discharge, and are attended by the hospital team, client and their family and the community team.

(Copyright: Stanmore IU Royal National Orthopaedic Hospital Trust 1996, with permission from the Spinal Injuries Unit)

Measurement of rehabilitation outcomes

in Box 6.4.

Rehabilitation needs to be measured not only in terms of disability but in terms of quality for the client. Lewinter and Mikkelsen (1995) carried out a small study in a stroke unit in Denmark, interviewing two occupational therapists, two nurses, two physiotherapists and one physician. The interviewees emphasised the importance of measuring quality in rehabilitation. They described quality as having physical/functional and social/normative dimensions. In the physical/functional dimension, they emphasised the difference in walking along a hospital corridor and walking to the corner shop. Quality in this dimension relates to overcoming normal physical barriers, for example, kerbs, roads, etc. The social/normative dimension was related to the fact that clients want to regain physical function but also want to be as 'normal' as possible. It can be stigmatising and isolating if the function clients regain is not seen as normal in other people's eyes, e.g. if they have problems with balance, or use a cumbersome walking aid.

Goal setting enables measurement to be at the level of quality for the client, comparing outcomes with the aims identified which should be at the level of handicap. By identifying objectives and targets which can be measured against time frames and against the overall aims, measurement can be quantitative with a qualitative element incorporating client's and family's comments.

Goal attainment scaling

Goal attainment scaling (GAS) developed by Kiresuk and Sherman (1968) has been used extensively to evaluate mental health programmes. GAS is a method which can be used to evaluate pre-established individual goals in order to assess the overall functioning of a service (Stanley, 1984) and to provide structure for objective documentation of clients' progress (Zweber and Malec, 1990).

GAS is a system of outcome measurement that involves the use of a 5-point scale. The long-term goal is identified and becomes point zero on the scale. Other levels of goal attainment are placed on the scale in reference to the long-term goal (Zweber and Malec, 1990). Although predominantly used in mental health care settings, GAS has been used in the evaluation of rehabilitation outcomes (Malec, Smigielski and De Pompole, 1991; Zweber and Malec, 1990: Grenville and Lyne, 1995). The following benefits of GAS in the rehabilitation setting have been identified in the literature:

- It provides structure to the goal setting meeting and provides a mechanism that encourages insight into the status and motivation of the client and their family (Zweber and Malec, 1990).
- It can assist in the development of the interdisciplinary team where interdisciplinary goal setting is paramount (Grenville and Lyne, 1995).
- It can facilitate the client's insight into problems being addressed in the rehabilitation programme (Zweber and Malec, 1990).

Discharge planning

Discharge planning is an essential part of the rehabilitation process. Planning needs to start as soon as the client is admitted. Planning should involve all relevant members of the team, the client and their family and professionals from the community.

Goal setting, with its focus on the level of handicap, can enhance the process of discharge by enabling clients and their families to focus on the roles in life they want to return to at the beginning of the rehabilitation programme. It should then become apparent what the expectations of the client and their family are regarding discharge. By involving clients and their families in the goal setting process from the beginning, and at the level of handicap, the team has the opportunity to prepare them to return to their community. The goal setting meetings themselves are opportunities to involve professionals from the community who need to be involved in the client's discharge process, e.g. the primary health care team. This will help bridge the gap in the interface between the ward or unit and the community.

The way forward

Goal setting in rehabilitation needs to be an interdisciplinary endeavor, which is a challenge for rehabilitation nurses. Whether it is possible to adopt such an approach will depend on their area of work. For example, on a medical ward it may not be possible, due to acute care taking priority over the implementation of a rehabilitation approach. However, the principles of goal setting and the issues around it as discussed do need to be taken on board if rehabilitation is to be effective.

Organisation of care

Rehabilitation nurses in general continue to organise their care using the principles of the nursing process, which is based on a biomedical approach to health care which is not congruent with a health promotion philosophy (Lindsey and Hartrick, 1996). As already discussed, interdisciplinary goal setting aims to promote empowerment which is a health promotion concept. Rehabilitation nurses may need to rethink the way they plan care, to ensure that it is congruent with an interdisciplinary approach. The nursing team at Rivermead Rehabilitation Centre in Oxford have gone through this rethinking process.

The primary nurses at Rivermead were finding that their nursing documentation and the way they planned care did not fit in with the unit's goal setting approach, which focused on impairment, disability and handicap. They tried to incorporate concepts such as empowerment, client choice, partnership and collaboration into the problem-solving approach of the nursing process. There was also incongruence between the goal setting approach and the nursing model they used which was an adapted form of Roper's activities of daily living model (Roper, 1976).

This change in thinking has resulted in the nursing documentation undergoing a number of changes, which has subsequently resulted in a change in the way nurses approach care planning. Difficulties for the client in the areas of disability and handicap are addressed in terms of focus, goal and evaluation. The documentation consists of a prompt sheet for the levels of disability and handicap. Rather than have headings on the nursing plans, the sheets are colour coded and the nurses use the prompt sheets to identify the areas of focus for the client (see Figure 6.2).

The next step is to use this new documentation for an agreed time and then evaluate the process. (This project is being led by E. Stone with input from A. Pill, S. Green, P. Briggs, T. Kinnersley and

Figure 6.2
Prompt sheets from the Rivermead Rehabilitation Centre, Oxford

Prompt Sheet
Rivermead Rehabilitation Centre, Oxford

(Disability = Pink)

1. **Washing and Dressing**
   How much help?
   Bath/shower
   Selecting clothes
   Washing/labelling

2. **Elimination**
   Menstruation
   Bladder/bowel
   (Vomiting)

3. **Eating and Drinking**
   Swallow/SALT
   Dental care
   Special diet
   Alcohol use
   Weight
   Appetite
   Likes/dislikes
   Allergies
   Food cut up

4. **Mobility**
   Pressure area care
   Transfers
   Safety
   Equipment
   Distance
   Stairs

5. **Sleep**
   Bed mobility
   Routine
   Safety

6. **Communication/Senses**
   Sight
   Speech
   Sensory/safety
   Hearing
   Foreign languages
   Aids

7. **Cognition and Perception**
   Visiospatial
   Sequencing
   Memory
   Concentration
   Problem-solving

8. **Social Conduct**
   Appropriate
   Impact on others
   Support system

9. **Pathology**
   Medication
   Diagnosis
   Relevant medical history
   Hereditary
   Pain

10. **Self-Concept**
    Sexuality
    Gender role
    Body image
    Self-esteem

11. **Adaptation to Self and Environment**
    Appropriate
    Impact on others
    Coping mechanisms
    Support systems

Figure 6.2a

Prompt Sheet
Rivermead Rehabilitation Centre, Oxford

(Handicap = Blue)

1. **Discharge Planning**
   Accommodation
   Lives with/pets
   Stairs
   Access
   Bathroom
   Kitchen skills
   Community skills
   Safety in the home
   Weekend leave
   Finances

2. **Support Network**
   Family
   Friends
   Colleagues/associates
   Formal/informal

3. **Work and Leisure**
   Finances
   Benefits
   Career aims
   Hobbies/interests
   Past/present/future

4. **Religion and Culture**
   Philosophy
   Place of worship
   Customs
   Beliefs
   Effect on past/present/future

Figure 6.2b

involvement from the nursing and interdisciplinary team.)

Other challenges that rehabilitation nurses need to consider to move forward are:

- **Client involvement.** How will clients and relatives be involved in the goal setting process? Obviously this also needs to be considered by the interdisciplinary team but nurses need to consider their role within the team and also as professionals.
- **Empowerment.** How will the principles of empowerment be promoted in nursing practice and what strategies will be used to ensure that these principles are consistent throughout the nursing team?
- **Consistency.** The nursing team will probably be the largest professional group within the interdisciplinary team and also the most diverse, with staff working different shifts, different hours and being at different levels of knowledge. It is a challenge for nurse managers in ensuring that all of the nursing team have the same understanding of the concepts related to goal setting and that they are all using the same approach.
- **Confidence.** Nurses need to feel confident in their own roles and not feel threatened where there is overlap of roles with other members of the interdisciplinary team. They also need to feel confident in taking on the additional roles associated with goal setting.

Conclusion

If the focus of rehabilitation is to be on the quality of life for an individual and not just on the minimising of impairment and disability, there need to be processes in place which enable this focus on handicap to happen. Interdisciplinary goal setting can be identified as being one of these processes. Goals set by nurses in isolation from the team and/or client will not fulfill the requirements of rehabilitation. Goal setting offers many challenges, not only to nurses but to all members of the team, and if these challenges can be met, the result will truly be an interdisciplinary team working with the client and their family in enabling the client to achieve their identified goals.

Questions for discussion

- What are the ethical issues related to goal setting?
- Have rehabilitation nurses got the skills to participate in interdisciplinary goal setting?
- How does the setting of nursing-specific goals fit into interdisciplinary goal setting?
- How can interdisciplinary goal setting be implemented in acute

hospital areas?

■ What is the role of nurses and other members of the team in promoting a philosophy of empowerment for clients and their families?

■ Is the way you organise your nursing care conducive with the philosophy of interdisciplinary goal setting?

References

Armentrout, G. (1993) A comparison of the medical model and the wellness model: the importance of knowing the difference. *Holistic Nurse Practitioner*, **7**, 57–62.

Caplan A. L. (1988) Informed consent and provider-patient relationships in rehabilitation medicine. *Archives of Physical Medical Rehabilitation*, **69**, 312–317.

Davis A., Davis S., Moss N., et al. (1992) First steps towards an interdisciplinary approach to rehabilitation. *Clinical Rehabilitation*, **6**, 237–244.

Dawson J & Bartlett E (1996) Change within interdisciplinary teamwork: one unit's experience. *British Journal of Therapy and Rehabilitation*, **3**, 219–222.

Embling S. (1995) Exploring multidisciplinary teamwork. *British Journal of Therapy and Rehabilitation*, **2**, 142–144.

Fugl-Meyer A. R., Branholm I. B. & Fugl-Meyer K. S. (1991) Happiness and domain-specific life satisfaction in adult northern Swedes. *Clinical Rehabilitation*, **5**, 25–33.

Galano J. (1977) Treatment effectiveness as a function of client involvement in goal setting and goal planning. *Goal Attainment Review*, **3**, 17–32.

Gibson C. H. (1991) A concept analysis of empowerment. *Journal of Advanced Nursing*, **16**, 354–361.

Golding L. & Allen P. (1990) Goal planning: a critical examination of its introduction into four houses in a London borough. *Mental Handicap*, **18**, 7–10.

Grenville J. & Lyne P. (1995) Patient-centred evaluation: *Journal of Advanced Nursing*, **22**, 965–972.

Hass J. (1993) Ethical considerations of goal setting for patient care in rehabilitation medicine. *Archives of Physical Medical Rehabilitation*, **72**, 228–232.

Ingram L. (1981) Effects of a home physical exercise program with a self-set goal on activity tolerance in chronic obstructive pulmonary disease. In *Proceedings of the Octoberquest, Research: The Nursing Frontier*, eds Roper J. & Hendrick E. Wadsworth CA: VA Medical Center.

Iveson C. (1994) Solution focused brief therapy: establishing goals and assessing competence: *British Journal of Occupational Therapy*, **57**, 95–98.

Jelles F., van Bennekom C. A. M. & Lankhorst G.J. (1995) The interdisciplinary team conference in rehabilitation medicine. *American Journal of Physical Medicine and Rehabilitation*, **74**, 464–465.

King I. M. (1981) *A Theory for Nursing*. New York: John Wiley.

Kiresuk T. & Sherman R. (1968) Goal attainment scaling: a general method of evaluating comprehensive mental health programmes. *Community Mental Health Journal*, **4**, 443–453.

Leddy S. & Pepper J. M. (1989) *Conceptual Bases of Professional Nursing*. Philadelphia: J. B. Lippincott Company.

Lewinter M. & Mikkelsen S. (1995) Therapists and the rehabilitation process after stroke. *Disability and Rehabilitation*, **17**, 211–216.

Lindsey E. & Hartrick G. (1996) Health-promoting nursing practice: the demise of the nursing process? *Journal of Advanced Nursing*, **23**, 106–112.

Locke E. A. (1968) Towards a theory of task motivation and incentives. *Organisational Behaviour and Human Performance*, **3**, 157–189.

Locke E. A. (1969) Purpose without consciousness: a contradiction. *Psychological Reports*, **25**, 991–1009.

Locke E. A., Shaw K. N., Saari L. M. & Latham G. P. (1981) Goal setting and task performance: 1969–1980. *Psychological Bulletin*, **90**, 125–152.

McGrath J. R. & Davis A. M. (1992) Rehabilitation:

where are we going and how do we get there? *Clinical Rehabilitation*, **6**, 225–235.

McGrath J. R. & Marks J. A. (1995) Towards inter-disciplinary rehabilitation: further developments at Rivermead Rehabilitation Centre. *Clinical Rehabilitation*, **9**, 320–326.

McGregor D. (1960) *The Human Side of Enterprise*. New York: McGraw Hill.

Malec J. F., Smigielski J. S. & DePompole R. W. (1991) Goal attainment scaling and outcome measurement in post acute brain injury rehabilitation. *Archives of Physical Medical Rehabilitation*, **72**, 138–143.

Malin N. & Teasdale K. (1991) Caring versus empowerment: considerations for nursing practice. *Journal of Advanced Nursing*, **16**, 657–662.

Manthey M. (1980) *The Practice of Primary Nursing*. London: Blackwell Scientific Publications Inc.

Maslow A. H. (1968) *Towards a Psychology of Being*, 2nd edn. Princeton, NJ: D Van Nostrand Reinhold.

Meichenbaum D. (1977) *Cognitive-Behaviour Modification*. New York: Plenum Press.

Naidoo J. & Wills J. (1994) *Health Promotion: Foundations for Practice*. London: Baillière Tindall.

Newell A. & Simon H. A. (1963) GPS a program that stimulates human thought. In *Computers and Thought*, Feigenbaum E. A., Feldman J., eds New York: McGraw Hill.

Price B. (1986) Giving the patient control. *Nursing Times*, **14**, 28–30.

Rodwell C. M. (1996) An analysis of the concept of empowerment. *Journal of Advanced Nursing*, **23**, 305–313.

Roper N. (1976) A model for nursing and nursology. *Journal of Advanced Nursing*, **1**, 219–227.

Schut H. A. & Stam H. J. (1994) Goals in rehabilitation teamwork. *Disability and Rehabilitation*, **16**, 223–226.

Smith R. & Draper P. (1994) Who is in control? An investigation of nurse and patient beliefs relating to control of their health care. *Journal of Advanced Nursing*, **19**, 884–892.

Stanley B. (1984) Evaluation of treatment goals: the use of goal attainment scaling. *Journal of Advanced Nursing*, **9**, 351–356.

Tyne A. (1994) Taking responsibility and giving power. *Disability and Society*, **9**, 249–254.

Urbanowski R. & Vargo J. (1994) Spirituality, daily practice, and the occupational performance model. *Canadian Journal of Occupational Therapy* **61** (2) 88–94.

van Bennekom, C. A. M., Jelles, F. & Lankhorst, G.J. (1995) Rehabilitation activities profile: the ICIDH as a framework for a problem – oriented assessment method in rehabilitation medicine. *Disability and Rehabilitation*.

Ventura M. R., Young D. E., Feldman M. J., Pastore P., Pikula S. & Yates M. A. (1983) Effectiveness of Health Promotion Interventions. *Nursing Research*, **33**, 162–167.

Wade D. T. (1996) *Rivermead Report Number Eight*. Oxford: Parchment (Oxford) Ltd.

World Health Organisation (1980) *International Classification of Impairment, Disabilities and Handicaps (ICIDH) a Manual of Classification*. WHO: Geneva.

Willer B. & Miller G. H. (1976) Client involvement in goal setting and its relationship to therapy outcome. *Journal of Clinical Psychology*, **32**, 687–690.

Zweber B. & Malec J. (1990) Goal attainment scaling in post-acute outpatient brain injury rehabilitation. *Occupational Therapy in Health Care*, **7**, 45–53.

Annotated further reading

King, I. M. (1994) Quality of life and goal attainment. *Nursing Quarterly*, **7**, 29–32.

This article explores King's theory of goal attainment in the promotion of health in relation to nursing.

Nicholson, J. R. (1984) Client centred rehabilitation: a method for setting realistic goals to meet client needs. *Journal of Rehabilitation*, **50**, 39–41, 72.

Schut, H. A. Stam, H.J. (1994) Goals in rehabilitation teamwork. *Disability and Rehabilitation*, **16**, 223–226.

Both of these articles explore the setting of realistic goals in rehabilitation settings.

Hass, J. (1993) Ethical considerations of goal setting for patient care in rehabilitation medicine. *American Journal of Physical Medicine and Rehabilitation*, **72**, 228–232.

This article explores the ethical considerations

and moral conflict that can occur when setting client goals.

Grenville, J. & Lyne, P. (1995) Patient-centred evaluation and rehabilitative care. *Journal of Advanced Nursing,* **22**, 965–972.

Issues surrounding outcome measurement in rehabilitative care discussing in particular the Barthel Index and Goal Attainment Scaling.

7 Delivering care

Kathy Bonney

Key issues
- Mode of care – the importance of empowerment in rehabilitation
- Skills of the rehabilitation nurse
- Delivering care in a rehabilitation setting
- Emotional and psychological barriers to rehabilitation

Introduction

The purpose of this chapter is to explore the issues surrounding care delivery within the area of rehabilitation nursing. It aims to inform the reader of how the nurse is able to deliver care as part of a multidisciplinary team. Many aspects of care are discussed, including specific problems associated with providing individualised client care within rehabilitation. The skills of the rehabilitation nurse are identified and explored, along with how the nurse complements other professionals within the team. Examples of how aspects of the client's life affect the rehabilitation process are included. The need to change the approach as different problems occur in order to succeed is discussed.

This chapter aims to examine the flexible approach required by rehabilitation nurses when they prescribe and deliver care. Skills required in rehabilitation may be the same as those required for other fields of nursing, however, it is the way these skills are applied in rehabilitation which makes the role of the rehabilitation nurse unique. There are also many barriers within rehabilitation which must be overcome if the client is to progress and reach their optimum level of ability.

Delivery of care means 'the way that nursing care is planned and put into practice', (Delivering Care, 1996a). The whole essence of delivering care within rehabilitation should focus on the clients and their family from the onset of illness. The way the care is organised is therefore determined by the needs of an individual. The rehabilitation nurse should provide a therapeutic environment with hope and encouragement for clients to reach their optimum level of ability. Goodwill (1990) insists that nursing the disabled client in hospital is a highly-skilled 'hands-off' process, where the nurse must encourage the patient to be as independent as possible.

Nurses caring for rehabilitation clients need to hold specialised knowledge and understanding of the rehabilitation process. Their skills should surpass these that were taught to them within their initial training. This is achieved through experience, education, and individual learning.

Rehabilitation nursing care can only be delivered effectively with support structures in place. These structures involve research, models and theories on which to base nursing practice, an interdisciplinary team approach for collaborative care planning and implementation, and a wider awareness of political and social issues surrounding the rehabilitation process.

Every client is entitled to the best care that can be provided, and the nurse who delivers that care must be fully committed to rehabilitation, and educated to a high standard within this field.

Mode of care

The needs of the client and the family will determine the level and type of care that is required. No two clients will require exactly the same care, although the initial nursing aims, to prevent complications and assist the client to become as independent as possible, should be paramount.

The rehabilitation nurse must offer constant support and positive reinforcement to the clients and their families from the beginning. At later stages of recovery this initial encouragement will help them to remain optimistic about their prognosis. Adams (1996) defines empowerment 'as the means by which the individuals . . . become able to take control of their circumstances and achieve their own goals, thereby being able to work towards helping themselves and others to maximise the quality of their lives'.

It is sometimes a difficult task, but the rehabilitation nurse must be able to empower the client so that they can start to take control of their lives again (see Case Study 7.1). It is also worth noting that there are clients who do not want to be empowered, and this must be respected. The level of difficulty in achieving empowerment depends on the client's own abilities. The aphasic client, for example, may have less chance of empowerment than somebody who can verbally express their wishes. Rehabilitation nurses must use their own communication skills effectively to ensure that client's own views are clearly represented:

Case study 7.1:
Client empowerment

Sarah is a 52 year old lady who had a cerebro-vascular accident only 3 years after the death of her husband. Together they had managed a business and looked after a plot of land which they rented out. Sarah's married daughter tried to persuade her to sell the land as nobody could look after it any longer.

Sarah refused.

The rehabilitation nurse was able to discuss the decision with Sarah. The social worker asked Sarah's daughter not to discuss the land with her, as the decision to sell had to come from Sarah. He explained to her about empowerment and the need for her mother to retain control over her life.

The understanding shown by the nurse when Sarah explained that the land was part of her life with her husband, assisted her to grieve. She was able to express the fact that, piece by piece, she felt that she was losing control of everything in her life.

After a few weeks, Sarah was able to discuss the land with her daughter again, this time asking her to sell it.

The decision had been Sarah's – she had lost control of many aspects of her life, but this had not been one of them.

The actual process of empowering a client may vary considerably with each individual, and the rehabilitation nurse should be aware of this. One of the best ways to empower a patient is to offer choice. Asking what a client would 'normally' prefer to do, and having the resources to carry out their wishes, is a positive step towards empowerment. Simply planning care with the client may be a method of empowerment, since the nurse is not dictating what is believed to be the best for the client. Another contributory factor towards empowerment may be the actual environment. If a client cannot find peace and quiet because there are no facilities to meet that need, then the client is given no choice. The rehabilitation nurse should include the client's own beliefs, wishes and goals in the delivery of care.

Empowerment may be of significant importance to a client who can no longer control their own body functions. They may be able to express how they would like to receive the care to meet those needs.

There is great skill involved in empowering the client. The first step is perhaps recognising that the client is experiencing powerlessness over their own life.

Skills of the rehabilitation nurse

The rehabilitation nurse needs to use many skills and techniques in order to deliver effective care. Some have already been identified, and others will now be examined. Rehabilitation nurses need to demonstrate a commitment to the speciality as well as a holistic approach to client care and a positive attitude.

The environment created needs to be conducive to rehabilitation, where 'normality' is encouraged. This may be done by creating a familiar environment with personal belongings in the client's room. The 'ward routine' needs to be tailored to the individual's own needs to allow them to establish their own patterns during the day. It is felt that some structure to the day is necessary for most clients; this may help a client identify with life before disability, where structures were in place, such as work. It may also assist clients to settle into this new environment when they first arrive.

Communicater

This skill is probably the most important one used within rehabilitation. The nurse needs to communicate effectively with many other people in many ways. Communication needs to be in a manner which is relevant to the actual circumstances, for example, the nurse may need to be calm, reassuring, assertive or understanding.

The nurse has a great deal of responsibility with regards to communication, such as the documentation of care plans. These are legal documents, and the nurse is responsible for clearly documenting prescribed care so that others can carry out that care.

Rehabilitation is a team effort and information needs to be shared. This can only be done through effective communication. Both formal and informal systems of communication should be in place (see Box 7.1).

Box 7.1

Example of communication strategies in rehabilitation

Rakehead Rehabilitation Centre, Burnley, Lancashire have developed the following strategies for communication:

- monthly formal meetings for heads of each discipline based at the centre
- monthly informal meetings for heads of each discipline based at the centre
- monthly formal meetings for rehabilitation nurses
- weekly team meetings for each primary therapy team to discuss their own clients; reviewing progress and goal planning
- weekly discussion meetings of all clients with the consultant and multidisciplinary team
- fortnightly discussion meetings between consultant, client and primary nurse (representing their own team members)
- monthly case conference for every client (or more or less often as required) involving the client, carers, consultant, multidisciplinary team members, and other agencies who may be involved, for example, district nurses
- collaborative care plans and evaluation documentation within one file
- diaries for each primary therapy team, for use of all staff
- display boards with names and addresses of organisations and associations around the centre
- leaflets on subjects surrounding rehabilitation and health promotion displayed around the centre
- Bi-monthly meeting for clients to express their views. This is called the SPEAC Group – satisfying patients by encouraging all to communicate

- carers' support group where there is the opportunity to express views
- suggestion box for clients and visitors
- individual pigeon holes for staff

However nurses communicate, it should always be clear and precise. It should always be checked that the person they are communicating with understands what is being said.

Listener

The skill to listen and not just hear takes time. The nurse must not only listen for small pieces of information which could indicate that clients have a problem they would like to share, but should also allow time for a client to express feelings. The rehabilitation nurse should liaise very closely with rehabilitation assistants (unqualified nursing staff), as the clients may be more likely to tell rehabilitation assistants information which is vital. This could be because rehabilitation assistants may seem less threatening to clients, and also because less formal relationships can be established.

Sometimes formal counselling is not required and a client may just benefit from expressing feelings to a nurse who has taken the time to listen. In fact, this time is well spent in preventing the need for formal counselling. The nurse must also listen carefully for signs that more formal counselling is necessary. Any doubts must be discussed with colleagues who may be able to meet that need.

Listening helps to build up trust and confidence in the nurse, leading to an open and honest relationship.

Facilitator

The nurse can help the client to accept that rehabilitation can be a slow process, by making it easier for them. This is done by setting achievable goals which offer direction for the client. As goals are achieved, they can then move forward with new ones. The nurse's ability to assist the client towards long-term goals is essential to prevent the client becoming frustrated and demotivated.

The rehabilitation nurse is a facilitator within the multidisciplinary team, ensuring that the different professionals and the clients are working towards common goals.

Enabler

As clients start to progress and achieve the goals they set with the nurse, they must know that the achievements are down to their own abilities. The nurse must guide clients so that they are empowered in decision-making, taking control over their own lives and accepting that the progress they are making is down to their own efforts. The knowledge that clients are responsible for their own achievements will help them to maintain the motivation to continue to strive for more independence.

The role of enabler varies considerably. The rehabilitation nurse may hold down a bread roll to enable the hemiplegic client to slice it and butter it, with the aim of becoming independent in this task. The rehabilitation nurse may also play a major part in enabling the client to make decisions about the care and treatment preferred. This is done simply by giving choice and not by dictating care. Lack of resources may have an impact on this however, and the rehabilitation nurse should make the most of the resources available. Even with limited resources, the rehabilitation nurse should be aware of clients' rights, such as those identified within the Patients' Charter, and these rights should be conveyed to the client.

If a client is dissatisfied with the care and treatment they are receiving, and if the problem cannot be resolved within the team, it is part of the nurse's role to enable the client to complain through the correct channels. Giving this information is important, not only to enable the client to do something to improve the service, but also within the role of advocate and empowerer, to give the client a voice.

Coordinator

As true rehabilitation needs the full cooperation of a multidisciplinary team, the nurse needs excellent coordination skills. Up to ten different disciplines can be involved in the care and treatment of an 'average' client, and for some, many more could be involved. Coordination of the team must be the role of the nurse who is there 24 hours-a-day, 7 days-a-week. This role needs a person who has excellent communication skills and a full understanding of the other roles involved. Different clinical management methods, such as primary nursing and keyworker systems, allow coordination to be easier because there are identified personnel involved with each patient. Time to coordinate the team should be allowed for, and formal meetings are essential.

At Rakehead Rehabilitation Centre in Burnley, Lancashire, for example, primary nursing is successful in facilitating effective communication. Its success may be due to the fact that each primary nursing team comprises a primary nurse, two associate nurses, three rehabilitation assistants, a physiotherapist, and an occupational therapist. All of these staff are named people who remain on the same team and treat the same group of clients. A named clinical assistant (doctor) covers two teams; there are four teams and two clinical assistants at the centre. The social worker and the speech and language therapist cover all four teams; both of these members of staff are also based at the centre. The rehabilitation nurse also coordinates the services of other professionals not based at the centre, but who are involved in the care and treatment of individuals on their team, such as the dietician or pharmacist.

Leader   The nurse's role as leader may be recognised or unrecognised. Either way, this is the nurse's role within the team. With a 24-hour picture of the client's activities and a greater insight into how the client is progressing, because of a holistic view, the client and the team can be helped towards common goals (see Case Study 7.2).

Case study 7.2:
Nurse as team leader

> The key rehabilitation nurse for Simon, a 29 year old, was informed that he had told the night nurse in charge he did not want to return home to his wife. The key nurse approached Simon, and he confirmed this was true. As the discharge date was pending, the nurse discussed alternative arrangements that Simon may be considering.
>
> He explained that he had nowhere else to go except to his parents home, on a temporary basis only. He wanted to live independently eventually. He told his nurse that he had spoken to his parents, and this had been agreed with them. His wife knew nothing of the decision at this point. His nurse explained that she would have to involve the other disciplines in order to assist Simon with his decision.
>
> The nurse firstly informed the social worker who was able to talk to Simon about his decision. He was also able to advise him to speak to his wife. At this stage, Simon refused the offer of marriage guidance counselling. However, the social worker offered to see the couple together if Simon required this.
>
> The nurse also called the multidisciplinary team involved in Simon's care to a meeting. This was purely to inform them of his decision. Once Simon had told his wife of his decision, a second meeting was called. This was to discuss Simon's discharge, and his future. He and his parents were in attendance. Home visits were planned and community staff involved.
>
> Simon was discharged to his parent's house only 2 weeks after his original discharge date. The social worker and community outreach team linked to the rehabilitation centre continued to see Simon post-discharge.
>
> He was eventually readmitted to the rehabilitation flat for a short period of time once a suitable home was found for him to live independently. Again, the social worker and community outreach team followed Simon home to help him to overcome problems he may encounter in his new home.

Collaborator   It is important to understand and respect the input from other disciplines. Collaborative care planning is believed to be essential in rehabilitation, where team members can work together with the client. Cooperation between disciplines is essential in order to meet the client's needs and reach planned outcomes. The nurse is in a position to identify problems at anytime during the client's rehabilitation, and collaboration with the other disciplines is essential to prescribe the best treatment and care. Good insight into the individual roles of other professionals is also essential if the rehabilitation nurse is to recognise needs from a therapy angle. Some of these needs may only be apparent when therapy staff are unavailable, such as at night. This emphasises the importance of 24-hour rehabilitation nursing. At Rakehead Rehabilitation Centre, there is a primary nursing system of rotation from days to nights using a set rota. This lends itself well to effective collaborative care planning, especially as therapy staff are part of the primary nursing teams.

Empowerer   Empowering a client can be a difficult process, where the nurse needs to demonstrate many skills to actually help the client to take control of their own circumstances. It may be necessary sometimes to obtain an independent advocate for the client if they require one. Time to see the clients is essential if they are to be effectively empowered.

Liaison   There need to be vital links to other services outside the rehabilitation unit to meet the client's needs. These may include services within the same hospital, or within the community. It is important to involve relevant services in case conferences if appropriate, so that the client can receive the services they require, especially if the service is required after discharge.

Rehabilitation nurses should not be afraid of involving specialist nurses, such as the stroke care nurse, with the client and family. Although their roles may be similar, both rehabilitation nurses and specialist nurses have different things to offer the client and family. They also complement each other with knowledge, and can support each other when dealing with complex needs and problems.

Advocate   Advocacy is described as 'more a matter of ensuring that no-one usurps the needs, rights and humanity of an individual' (Delivering Care, 1996b). The nurse needs to support the client throughout their rehabilitation. This process may involve empowering the client to use information obtained by the nurse in order to overcome problems or obstacles. The nurse should be responsive to clients' rights and have access to organisations which may be able to assist. Many areas offer an advocacy service which is free to the client. It is the nurses' role, with the multidisciplinary team, to ensure that the client is represented. Nurses do, to some degree, take this role on board, but it is usually with the less complex decisions such as day-to-day requirements. Rehabilitation nurses may be asked to challenge the treatment prescribed by another professional on behalf of the client.

It does not usually, however, come to this if there is effective communication and interdisciplinary working. However, the client should be represented and the skillful rehabilitation nurse should be able to do this without jeopardising relationships with colleagues. There may also be policies in place to support the nurse in their role as advocate. For example, a policy for the protection of vulnerable adults is used at Burnley Health Care in Lancashire, to inform staff how to recognise various forms of abuse, such as physical, sexual, financial, legal, emotional and psychological. As client advocate, the rehabilitation nurse can use the policy to protect the client.

Educator

It is the nurse's role to educate not only the client, but the family, carers and other staff. This will involve rehabilitation techniques, prevention of complications, promotion of a healthy lifestyle and other aspects surrounding disability. The nurse will act as a resource for information and clarification. The appropriate knowledge and skills will be passed to the relevent people throughout the rehabilitation programme. There are many ways of educating people, and all should be considered to give information. The rehabilitation nurse may use any of the techniques in Box 7.2 to educate another person. The list is not comprehensive.

Box 7.2
Educational techniques

- Informal teaching sessions, either one-to-one or within groups.
- Formal teaching sessions, usually used for staff training rather than client/carer education.
- Leaflets offering information in brief.
- Booklets offering information in more detail on chosen subjects.
- Demonstrations, for example, how to apply a urinary sheath.
- Videos, for example, on health promotion issues.
- Photographs, for example, of a person's own pressure sore to demonstrate how tissue can break down if pressure relief is not maintained.
- Books and journals, for both staff and clients. Files on certain aspects of care are a useful resource to have available for easy reference.
- Other professionals, for example, from The Stroke Association, to educate staff, clients and carers on particular aspects relevent to certain conditions.
- Courses for staff, either 'in-house' with input from other disciplines, or external courses.
- Working in collaboration with the multidisciplinary team. This is particularly useful to educate staff on individual clients.

Planner

Not only is the nurse planning short-term goals alongside the client and other professionals, but also long-term goals. Discharge planning, for example, should be evident throughout the rehabilitation programme. In this case, planning involves others, such as community agencies. It is essential to plan with all relevent disciplines so that possible problems may be prevented. The planning process should be ongoing, and the rehabilitation nurse should be prepared to accept changes to planned programmes as a normal part of rehabilitation.

Case study 7.3:
Rehabilitation nurse as planner

> After 4 months of rehabilitation, Susan had accepted that she was unable to care for her husband, Jim, at home. It had been a heart-breaking decision for this young woman whose husband was both physically and cognitively impaired. She had received support from her family, and also from staff at the rehabilitation centre.
>
> At the case conference where discharge planning was being concluded, Susan was asked if she had been able to make any decisions from the information given to her about Jim's preferred place of discharge. At this point, Susan stated that she wanted Jim to be discharged to their own home.
>
> The consultant then discussed some of the problems Susan and Jim may encounter with this decision. He also reiterated the reasons why Susan had come the the decision that she would not manage her husband at home. Although Susan said she understood the implications, she still wanted to know how feasable this could be.
>
> The rehabilitation nurse then informed those present at the case conference that a study would commence to determine the level of input Jim required from both qualified and unqualified nursing staff. This would help identify the care package requirements, and, of course the funding required to discharge Jim to his own home. Susan was also invited to stay for periods of time in the rehabilitation flat with her husband, both during the week when she worked, and also at the weekend when she did not.
>
> This change in plan to Jim's rehabilitation programme enabled Susan to finally accept that her husband would need 24-hour nursing input for the foreseeable future.

Consultant

The rehabilitation nurse within their own field will act as a resource for clients, families, carers, and other nursing and therapy staff. This is part of the role not only whilst the client is in the rehabilitation unit, but prior to admission and post-discharge. It may be likely that the nurse's opinion is sought from staff caring for the client prior to admission to the rehabilitation centre. Sometimes staff within other fields of nursing may simply require confirmation that their approach is the right one.

Researcher   The rehabilitation nurse not only uses research findings, but also contributes to research. It is ensured that research is disseminated to the team and used to benefit the client. Researched-based practice can also be used to assist clients in making their own decisions and choices in their care. They can be presented with the facts, which will hopefully ensure that the clients choose the best options available. The research can also be used by the nurse as a tool to help persuade the client that they need to do certain tasks, for example, in relation to pressure relief.

Rehabilitation nurses should focus very much on research because, no matter what the client's diagnosis is, there should be a consistent approach using the rehabilitation process. Problems can occur when different approaches are used, possibly because of each individual nurse's preference (for example in wound care), and this could hinder a client's rehabilitation and certainly prolong their length of stay in hospital. Rehabilitation is a long enough process without introducing complications which could prevent an earlier discharge from hospital.

Delivering care in a rehabilitation setting

Roper, Logan and Tierney (1983) based their nursing model on activities of daily living, and this model can be used as a framework upon which to plan care within the rehabilitation setting. This model is well recognised and commonly used in many fields of nursing. Aspects particular to rehabilitation nursing care required for each of these activities of daily living are discussed below.

Physical aspects   *Maintaining a safe environment*

The rehabilitation of a client should commence at the onset of illness. Maintaining a safe environment is vital in any field of nursing, but within rehabilitation, the environment can have a positive or negative effect on the client's recovery. An example of this might be the correct assessment and use of aids to help the client into and out of the bath without risk. The rehabilitation nurse should educate clients to be aware of their own limitations.

Communication   At all stages of the rehabilitation process, effective communication is vital. Within rehabilitation, it is important to keep the client orientated to time and place. Non-verbal communication is also important. To communicate effectively, it is essential that the nurse works closely with the client, the family, and the speech and language therapist if there are actual speech problems. Appropriate communication methods must be used consistently by all nursing staff for each individual. The nurse's role is also to facilitate communication between clients and their relatives/visitors by demonstrating any aids/equipment used or discussing the best ways of communicating.

The importance of communication in rehabilitation can relate to being able to keep the client informed of their progress, which in turn may assist in motivating them to achieve more.

Breathing   Whalley-Hammell (1995) states that 'regular turning prevents stasis of secretions in dependent areas of the lungs . . . and even minor changes of position will prevent accumulation of secretions'. This is a part of rehabilitation nursing: prevention of complications. Their role as educator for the client who smokes may also be vital in helping to prevent further illness. Close liaison with the physiotherapist at this stage is important.

Eating and drinking   Goodwill and Chamberlain (1990) suggest that, 'the patient's morale is considerably improved when he is able to eat and drink independently with as little mess as possible'. The rehabilitation nurse must try to encourage 'socially acceptable' feeding with clients seated together within a dining room. This is a normal part of life for many people, usually with the family or when eating out socially. Simple advice, such as drinking from cups that are only half-full, or using a straw for clients who are ataxic, can help with independence and self-confidence. Careful positioning at the table can assist in self-feeding, and prevent choking episodes. Simply having serviettes available for clients to wipe their own mouths can help them to feel more comfortable when eating with others. Goodwill and Chamberlain identify meal times as being a good opportunity to improve social skills, with clients being invited to help set and clear tables. This is a small but useful step towards independent living for some clients.

It is the nurse's role to liaise with the dietitian to establish diet and fluid intake to meet the nutritional needs of each individual client. Close liaison with the speech and language therapist is important for the dysphagic patient.

Elimination   The holistic approach used by rehabilitation nurses, whereby all aspects of a client's life are addressed, enables them to fully understand the importance of elimination for a client. The most influencial aspects regarding the maintainance of elimination are a healthy diet, good fluid intake and exercise. These are the areas the nurse should focus on and adjust where necessary.

The aim is to maintain urinary continence so that the client can lead a normal life. Liaison with the continence advisor may help to determine the correct way of preventing, or at least reducing, incontinence. As there are different types of incontinence, each client will benefit from different regimes. The nurse's role is to implement that regime and support the client in a positive manner.

Urinary sheaths for men who are incontinent are a possibility and the nurse must teach the client himself how to apply the sheath, if appropriate. If this is not possible, then a relative or carer can be taught to do this.

Catheters are sometimes the only alternative for women and some men, where incontinence cannot be managed in any other way. Dangers of infection must be explained, along with other potential complications such as the tube becoming blocked. It is the nurse's role to ensure that these problems are prevented, and educating the client properly is the first step in prevention. The client must be fully aware of signs and symptoms of these problems and the action they must take if they occur.

One of the more acceptable methods of preventing incontinence is self-catheterisation. Whalley-Hammell (1995) states that:

> *'Individuals who catheterise themselves may use a clean method rather than sterile technique, although many sources recommend a sterile procedure while in hospital because of the high risk of contamination'.*

It is important that the nurse does not dissuade the client from self-catheterisation by stressing the importance of sterility whilst in hospital. Instead, the benefits should be highlighted to the client. According to Whalley-Hammell, these include freedom from an external collecting device, reduced risks of infection and calculi, enhanced sexual relations, and improved personal hygiene (especially for women).

Technique demands some manual dexterity, and the nurse must ensure the client is given all the support necessary to feel comfortable with their technique.

The inability to control the bowel can also create serious problems if not managed properly. It is of extreme importance that a thorough assessment of the client's normal lifestyle and habits takes place. Everyone is an individual, with individual bowel regimes.

Personal cleansing and dressing

The rehabilitation nurse's role in this area of care is to assist the client in becoming as independent as possible. Motivating the client to want to be independent is sometimes the more difficult obstacle to overcome, as tasks which were once taken for granted can be quite difficult to manage with a disability. It is important that the nurse acknowledges how clients may feel when assistance is required with hygiene and dressing. It is possible the client may feel like a child, and efforts to maintain privacy and dignity should be made at all times.

For the client who is completely dependent on the nurse in the early stages of illness, it may be more acceptable for the nurse to fulfil this role. Turnbull and Bell (1985) agree that during the acute phase it is important that strategies which will complement later rehabilitation efforts should be implemented. They continue to stress that the nurse in an acute setting needs to be well aquainted with rehabilitation concepts and procedures.

Even at this stage, the rehabilitation nurse should be looking at the client's potential abilities and identifying small goals. It should be second nature for a rehabilitation nurse to involve the client in their care, and what may seem like minor achievements, such as a client holding a cloth to their face whilst the nurse washes their hair, are major steps to reaching that optimum level of ability. The nurse will observe these small improvements and use them as a base to build on. As clients achieve goals they will feel inspired to attempt the next step. It is essential to set very realistic goals that will be achieved, and especially to encourage clients to set their own. All disciplines should be involved in goal setting to enable the client to reach their full potential. Goal planning is explored in Chapter 6.

Close liaison with the occupational therapist is essential to identify correct techniques in hygiene and dressing for each individual. As the rehabilitation nurse is there 24 hours a-day, 7 days-a-week, these techniques must be implemented every single time the client is washing, dressing or undressing. Evaluation of their progress should be monitored closely and fed back to the occupational therapist. It is important that the nurse and therapist work together so that the client recognises that the treatment is continuing whether the occupational therapist is there or not. Goodwill and Chamberlain (1990) states that a client feels better if dressed in normal clothing rather than nightclothes and that, as far as possible, practice in regaining this skill should be given at the correct time of day.

Two contributing factors to the client accepting these tasks are choice and time. It is important that the nurse recognises the client's individuality and accepts these choices where possible. These may include choice of hygiene facilities, time of preferred wash/bath/shower, choice of clothes, etc. The time element is essential – for true rehabilitation, time must be available for the client to achieve their goal. Alongside personal cleansing and dressing are other issues associated with appearance, such as hairstyle and make-up. Clients sometimes need a lot of encouragement to take pride in their appearance as they did before.

Controlling body temperature

Some clients may have physiological problems with controlling body temperature. Strategies to maintain a comfortable body temperature should be discussed, such as increasing the level of fluid intake. Also the client must learn to recognise when something is wrong, for example, feeling very hot could be an indication of infection. The dangers of being unable to control body temperature may apply to certain clients.

Whalley-Hammell (1995) discusses clients with spinal cord injuries who are susceptible to both heat prostration and hypothermia due to major impairments of the body's ability to modify heat production and loss. The normal way to become warmer may be to get closer to the electric fire, but the dangers to a client who has lost sensation include severe burns.

Clients must be taught to think more carefully about what they do and the consequences of their actions.

Mobilising
Mobilising is interrelated to all other activities of living. Being unable to mobilise independently is the biggest problem for many clients. The environment can sometimes play a big part in either helping or hindering a client's mobility. Goodwill and Chamberlain (1990) provide examples by saying that cold, uninviting, inaccessible areas will not encourage 'wheelchair independence'. They also mention the lack of rails which, again, reduce the ability for some clients to mobilise independently.

In the acute stages of illness, it is essential that problems associated with immobility are prevented. The list is endless, but the more serious problems include chest infection, deep-vein thrombosis which could lead to pulmonary embolism, pressure sores and spasticity.

The nurse must work closely with the physiotherapist to establish correct moving and handling techniques and best positions to nurse the client in. Passive exercises may be necessary and change of position is essential to prevent complications. Turnbull and Bell (1985) support this and explore the rehabilitation nurse's educational role. They discuss 'Bobath' techniques (based on the principles of normal movement), which are still encouraged, and stress an integral part of the re-education process as being the actual concept of symmetry of the body and limbs. There may be a combination of problems, such as muscle weakness, spasticity, incoordination and sensory loss, which will need individual treatment (Goodwill and Chamberlain, 1990).

For the hemiplegic patient, it is essential that the nurse positions tables, lockers and other sources of interest to the patient's affected side. Turnbull and Bell (1985) explore the advantages of this. The rehabilitation nurse needs to be aware of these advantages to increase their own self-awareness and to enable them to educate carers and visitors.

The advantages in positioning things to the affected side are:

- It minimises the tendency to ignore the affected side.
- It stimulates the client to the environment on their affected side.
- It encourages the client to look and reach towards the affected side.
- It promotes weight-bearing through their affected hip.
- it reduces abnormal muscle tone by rotation of the spine.
- it prevents the patient from compensating for the paralysis.
- if there is a visual field deficit, the client is encouraged to turn the head.

Turnbull and Bell (1985) continue to discuss the importance of correct positioning to encourage 'normal body image' through proper body alignment. Support aids, such as arm rests for the affected arm, can be useful in the prevention and reduction of oedema, and other aids, such as a collar and cuff have been known to help prevent subluxation of the shoulder (it is important to note that a collar and cuff used for the prevention of subluxation has been recently recognised to have most benefit by increasing awareness of the affected shoulder). It is important to liaise closely with the physiotherapist when considering positioning.

Comfort is also important and the nurse must encourage the client to do as much as possible to alter their own position. This will help increase sensation and stimulation of the affected side.

Special mattresses or beds may be required depending on the assessment of each individual client. Liaison with the tissue viability nurse is useful. Problems must be prevented, for once something goes wrong, such as the client developing a deep-vein thrombosis, rehabilitation will be more difficult. It is important for the nurse to be fully aware of the signs and symptoms of these potential problems in the early stages, so that damage can be avoided or at least minimised.

Once clients start to recover from the acute stage of their illness they should be encouraged and assisted to mobilise as much as they can independently. Sometimes, however, it may be necessary to limit mobility, for example, for somebody with multiple sclerosis to conserve energy. The rehabilitation nurse can monitor the client's level of mobility over 24 hours, and throughout that period, varying degrees of assistance may be required. A client who can stand and transfer in the morning may need assistance in the evening. Risk assessments relating to mobility are essential to prevent injury to the client and the nurse.

Helping a client to accept reduced mobility can be difficult. The nurse must focus on positive achievements, particularly smaller movements which allow the client independence in certain tasks.

Again, the client must be educated on the dangers of immobility and how to prevent these from occurring.

Working and playing

Disability may initially prevent the patient from working. This could also prevent 'play', as the two are interrelated. Many people work in order to earn money. As Goodwill and Chamberlain (1990) suggest, while money does not solve disability, lack of it certainly compounds the problem. The nurse's role, with the team, is to help the clients to come to terms with their disability and to accept that they cannot return to the lifestyle they had before in relation to work and play. Outside advice and support can be obtained from professionals specifically involved with employment, and the client must be made aware of the options available. This could be modifying the work into an alternative occupation. Close liaison with the social worker is necessary so that the problem of financial loss can be minimised with knowledge of benefit entitlements.

Many people believe their life is over if they cannot contribute to their family and society. It is important that the nurse focuses on the client's abilities. Skills acquired through work and hobbies can be redirected to something constructive during a rehabilitation programme. Finding a person's likes and dislikes can lead to new developments and creative ideas. There may be certain ventures that a client would have liked to pursue, but never had the time before because of work commitments. These opportunities may include art, literature, sport or other specific interests. The interests must be realistic and the support must be available. It is essential to help the client to prevent boredom, and to gain satisfaction from achieving new challenges (see Case Study 7.4).

Case study 7.4:
Working and playing

> Tom is a 47 year old computer specialist who, prior to his stroke, worked 7 days a week for up to 12 hours a day. He earned over £4000 a month and rarely saw his family. His whole life changed significantly when he had his stroke. He saw his family every day, he learned how to cook, he met new people, he wrote poetry, he helped others by reading to them, he devised a computer programme, he booked a holiday...
>
> The rehabilitation nurses assisted in Tom's change in lifestyle by encouraging him to focus on his abilities, and how his skills might be put to good use in a different setting.
>
> Whereas Tom could only see what he had lost, the rehabilitation nurses enabled him to see what he had actually gained.

Resources such as computers are sometimes required to help clients regain skills. If the ward or rehabilitation unit does not have these facilities, then clients should be assisted to bring their own things in.

Expressing sexuality

Roper, Logan and Tierney (1983) found that most people associated sexuality with sexual intercourse, even though intercourse is only a small part of sexuality. Unfortunately, nurses often ignore this aspect of a client's life and concentrate on other areas of their sexuality during assessment. The way in which individuals dress, act and communicate are all areas that reflect their sexuality. Webb (1985) supports this, saying that people are sexual beings all of the time, whether they are healthy, ill or disabled, and they express their sexuality in unique, individual ways. The continuation of this individualised behaviour is important so that the client still has that same identity as before. The nurse must encourage this to continue so that the client feels as much the same as possible. This will help to maintain relationships already established in life. Close observation is required to see how clients interact with other people, especially those closest to them.

It is important that clients with partners maintain their previous relationship if both people wish to do so. It is easy to fall into a patient/carer relationship which can bring untold problems if those are not the preferred roles. Some of these problems stem from feelings. These may include guilt, resentment, frustration, pity, disgust and loneliness. Goodwill and Chamberlain (1990) comment that 'lack of understanding' of sexuality and the problems associated with it, will compound any other problems. He discusses 'poor self-image', feelings of being 'incomplete' or 'damaged', which impairs psychological and sexual function as well as every other aspect of their life. That relationship needs to be secure to lead back to practicalities involving physical relationships. Patients and their partners must feel comfortable talking about their sexual relationships, and it is very often the nurse they will turn to for advice. Newton (1991) discusses simple pieces of advice, such as modifying sexual activity and conserving energy. The nurse may be able to offer advice to the client, but other resources which may be helpful should be available. These could be other staff who have undergone training, or special organisations which deal specifically with sexual problems relating to disability. As this is a very 'taboo' subject for many clients, the nurse must listen for tiny hints that advice is sought. For those who do not indicate that advice is sought, information such as leaflets and other resources such as named members of staff who have undergone further training should be available. The service should be available for partners of clients also. Introduction of the subject of sex could simply be in the form of an informative leaflet given to the client to read.

Nurses must also observe for inappropriate sexual behavior, sometimes directed at themselves. It is important that behaviour is acceptable within society as a person could be ostracised if they do not conduct themselves in the 'normal' way. The cause could be pathological, such as with brain injury, and it is therefore important to reeducate a person regarding socially acceptable behaviour. Another reason may be frustration or an attempt to 'prove' a client's man- or womanhood still exists. This needs to be dealt with firmly and sensitively with the support of appropriate colleagues. It can happen with both men and women equally.

Sleeping   Sleep is an extremely important part of rehabilitation because the body cannot function without it. If the client has enough sleep (the amount of which varies from person to person) then the activities carried out when awake will be much easier to fulfil. The rehabilitation nurse must try to establish as near the normal sleep pattern as possible for the client, and help to maintain that. The pattern could be affected by many things, the main one being a different environment when in hospital. The client can only be assessed once settled into the new environment.

If the sleep pattern is disturbed then the nurse and client must discuss the reasons for not sleeping. Some of the problems can possibly be eliminated straight away, for example, by reducing excess noise or light. Other problems may take more time, such as reassuring clients about their worries. Some clients simply lose their normal sleep pattern through having a sleep during the day. The reasons must be identified.

Evaluation of sleep must be communicated to other disciplines who may help, for example, occupational therapy could include relaxation techniques as part of treatment.

All avenues to promote normal sleep must be explored. Medical intervention and drug therapy may be necessary, but this should only ever be a short-term measure.

Dying This is included because 'the process of living is a fatal one and the final act of living is dying'. Every nurse hopes to care for the dying patient in a way that prevents pain and suffering, leading to a peaceful and dignified death. The comforting of loved ones during and after the client's death is vital.

For the client who is ill, dying can be a real fear, even though it may not be imminent.

The nurse should try to allay these fears, and good communication is vital. Sometimes, clients may feel they want to die because they see their life being over if they are left with a permanent disability. The key role here is to promote a positive outlook on life and once again focus on ability, health and wellness.

Emotional and psychological aspects All of the physical activities of living can be affected by the client's emotional state. The illness can create many feelings which may be predominantly negative. It is the role of the rehabilitation nurse and the whole team to assess these feelings (which may change often), explore them and try to help the client control or come to terms with them. This is not always possible as the client may not show their true feelings to any member of staff. Involvement from other disciplines is vital and good communication between keyworkers is essential.

The care the nurse delivers will depend on the emotional and psychological well being of the client, as well as the physical needs. It is the nurse's role to understand and accept these needs. According to Dittmar (1989) the following goals should be mutually established with the client and their family:

- to maintain or restore self-esteem
- to maintain or restore ability to perform activities of living
- to maintain or restore role functions within the family network
- to obtain emotional support during the adjustment to the disability
- to express grief
- to openly communicate within the family network
- to accomplish social adjustment goals
- to use the expertise of rehabilitation team members as necessary.

Some of the feelings associated with these goals are discussed below, with the care required by the rehabilitation nurse.

Anxiety   Anxiety and illness are often associated with each other. Anxiety can be reduced in many ways, such as simply welcoming the client to the ward, and introducing key staff. Communication is probably the best way of allaying fears associated with being in hospital. Opportunities to discuss issues which may cause anxiety should be given, and it is important that the nurse builds up a good rapport with the client to facilitate good communication.

Depression   True clinical depression needs full medical treatment, probably including anti-depressants, and specialist psychiatric input. For the rehabilitation nurse within a nonpsychiatric setting, it is sometimes difficult to fully understand the mind of a depressed person. Stewart (1985) suggests that the feelings of depression may 'last for years', with a continuous 'helpless feeling'.

However, as the rehabilitation nurse acknowledges this condition, she can adjust the delivery of care accordingly. It is usual for a client who is depressed to lack the motivation to be rehabilitated, so the team must try and adjust the programme to facilitate this. Communication with the client is vital in order to ascertain how much the client is able to contribute. Positive reinforcement is also important, offering the client realistic goals. Close observation of mood and behaviour is essential to give feedback to other professionals who will be counselling the client.

Sometimes clients who are not 'depressed' can become 'low in mood'. It is at this stage that, firstly, the nurse must recognise this emotional state and then focus on positive aspects of a client's care and progress to date. It is also essential for the client to be allowed to express feelings – sometimes they may just need to talk through their feelings with a nurse.

It is of vital importance that the nurse recognises when a client appears depressed and withdrawn, for the possibility of a suicidal client cannot be ignored, and greater expertise is then required.

Grieving   The loss of a body part, function or control over one's own activities can lead to feelings of deep sorrow. The nurse must accept these feelings and assist the client to go through the stages of grief. Hafen and Frandsen (1983) believe that experiencing grief is necessary, because without it, healing cannot take place. The stages of grief as identified by Engel (1964), and the nurse's role within each stage are identified below.

The first stage of grief is shock and disbelief. It is hard for a person to accept disability and the easiest way to cope with this is through denial. The reality is not emotionally recognised and the client may feel numb. The nurse must observe for this first sign, which could be shown in different ways. One such way is for the client to keep 'busy' with hospital routines and visitors. This allows the client to avoid true feelings by pushing them to one side. This stage can last any amount of time, from minutes to days. The nurse must spend time with the client to allow the start of acceptance of the disability, and residual abilities.

Stewart (1985) suggests that it is difficult at this stage to make 'emotional contact'. He continues to state that clients 'are usually unwilling to accept the abnormality, do not wish to hear treatment plans which do not include a cure and return to pre-morbid stage, and often go from physician to physician accepting therapies which give promise of a cure'.

Awareness follows, once the client has realised that there are disabilities, and feelings may be expressed about this in different ways. Again, the nurse must recognise these feelings as part of the grieving process. They may be expressed in anger, frustration or bitterness towards others. Time spent with the client and showing an understanding of their feelings will help them through this stage. Allowing the client to express these feelings is vital, so they may shout and scream, or cry. It is important to be there for the client to vent these feelings. Feelings of anger could be directed inward, toward the client, or outward. Stewart (1985) recognises that it could be outward 'to others' or just 'toward life itself'. The nurse must be aware, as Stewart states, that the anger could be 'destructive if it is prolonged to the point where it antagonises those who would try to help but who feel constantly repelled by it'.

After awareness comes restitution. The disability is more real to the client at this stage, as friends and relatives gather round to share the loss. The fact that others are there to lend support encourages the client to try and take control of their life again. Once some degree of control is regained, the client feels less helpless.

Goodwill and Chamberlain (1990) suggest that 'a disabled person disables the family, to some degree limiting their choice in life'. He continues to remind us that 'a disabled person has duties as well as rights; the same as any other member of the family'. The nurse should encourage the client to take up as much of their previous life as is possible, and to develop new interests with a life 'outside'. Indeed, this may be an objective of the client's rehabilitation.

Resolution occurs as the client adjusts to their individual loss. The achievement of small goals may act as a motivator to achieve bigger goals. The team plays a key role at this stage in helping the client to set the goals and achieve them. The nurse must focus on all positive achievements and recognise the client's own limits. Stewart describes this stage as being 'prepared to accept the disability'.

All of these emotional feelings can be barriers to a successful rehabilitation programme. It is essential that emotional and psychological aspects of a person's life are embraced as a normal part of the rehabilitation process.

Conclusion

As rehabilitation nurses, it is essential that we embrace various concepts and theories in the care we prescribe and the approach we take. The degree of skill, knowledge and attitude needed to deliver care in a rehabilitation setting is extremely high, as there are many obstacles to overcome.

The client may need to change their whole lifestyle, especially if there is permanent disability. Within the 'safety' of a rehabilitation centre, this may not be too difficult to accept, so the emphasis should be on the client's life once they have left the centre. It would be easy for the nurse to over-sympathise with the client and family, but this will only delay the rehabilitation process. The ability to understand the client and how their life will be affected is much more constructive, because the nurse can then help plan the best ways to overcome the obstacles met.

If holistic care is to be delivered, then all parts of care must be analysed as each affects the other. All aspects of a client's lifestyle must be addressed, because otherwise, the rehabilitation programme will not be complete. The family should be involved from the beginning so that their own problems and fears can be explored.

The rehabilitation nurse is the lynch-pin in the programme of care. There must be a view of the client's life before the onset of illness, during the period of rehabilitation at the centre, and post-discharge. The client should leave a rehabilitation programme with direction and the motivation to continue to strive for goals throughout life.

Questions for discussion

- When should rehabilitation nursing commence?
- What factors should be considered regarding the vast amount of time needed to deliver care in a rehabilitation setting?
- What differences are there between rehabilitation nursing and other specialities?
- What skills are required by rehabilitation nurses?
- How should a rehabilitation nurse deal with a client who has lost the motivation to progress further?

- Who should set the goals for individual clients?

- How is the effect of the delivery of care measured?

- Why is client empowerment important in rehabilitation?

- How do other professionals influence the delivery of rehabilitation nursing care?

- What is the importance of communication within rehabilitation?

References

Adams, R. (1993) *Social Work and Empowerment*, 2nd edn. London: MacMillan Press.

Campbell, D. & Spence A.A. (1983) *A Nurse's Guide to Anaesthetics, Resuscitation and Intensive Care*, 7th edn. London: Churchill Livingstone.

Delivering Care (1996a) 1 – Delivery Systems. *Professional Nurse*, **11**, 459–463.

Delivering Care (1996b) 2 – Conflicts in care. *Professional Nurse*, **11**, 529–532.

Dittmar, S. (1989) Rehabilitation Nursing – Process and Application. St. Louis: C.V. Mosby Co.

Goodwill, J.C. & Chamberlain, M.A. (1990) *Rehabilitation of the Physically Disabled Adult.* London: Chapman and Hall.

Newton C. (1991) *Roper, Logan and Tierney Model in Action.* London: MacMillan.

Roper, N., Logan, W.W. & Tierney, A.J. (1983) *Using a Model for Nursing.* Edinburgh: Churchill Livingstone.

Stewart, W. (1985) *Counselling in Rehabilitation.* London: Croom Helm.

Turnbull, G.I. & Bell P.A. (1985) *Maximising Mobility After Stroke – Nursing the Acute Patient.* London: Croom Helm.

Webb C. (1985) *Sexuality, Nursing and Health.* London: HM & M.

Whalley-Hammell, K., (1995) *Spinal Cord Injury Rehabilitation.* London: Chapman and Hall.

Annotated further reading

Delivering Care, Part 1 (1996) Delivery systems. *Professional Nurse*, 1996, **11**, 459–463.

Delivering Care, Part 2 (1996) Conflicts in care. *Professional Nurse*, 1996, **11**, 529–532.

Delivering Care, Part 3 (1996), Working in a team. *Professional Nurse*, 1996, **11**, 601–605.

Delivering Care, Part 4 (1996), Managing a team. *Professional Nurse*, 1996, **11**, 679–682.

This series examines methods of delivering care to clients. The first part covers 'Delivery Systems' such as task allocation, team nursing, primary nursing and multidisciplinary team care. The second examines assertiveness, accountability, ethics and advocacy. Part three defines 'teamwork' and explores types, roles and motivation. Finally, part four includes leadership skills, delegation, and other aspects of managing a team.

Royal College of Nursing 1991 *The Role of the Nurse in Rehabilitation of Elderly People.* London: Scutari Press.

In this document rehabilitation is explored 'in its widest context'. It includes philosophy and definitions of rehabilitation and old age. It explores the profile of the elderly population and the needs of elderly people. It identifies aspects of the nurse's role in rehabilitation. Brief discussion of constraints within rehabilitation also takes place.

Porritt, L. (1984) *Communication: Choices for Nurses.* Edinburgh: Churchill Livingstone.

This book provides an overview of the process of communication and factors contributing to its ineffectiveness or effectiveness, with regard to verbal and non-verbal aspects. It discusses the importance of how varying interpretations of what is communicated can impact on how we interact with others. It also discusses the skills required to be an effective communicator.

Brown, R. I., Bayer M. B. (1992) *Empowerment and Development Handicaps: Choices and Quality of Life.* London: Chapman & Hall.

This book includes a report of a 6-year study in western Canada. The objectives were to see how individuals progressed, to observe their lives and to measure performance in a range of vocational, social and educational areas. It identified the need for the group to develop more assertiveness, higher motivation, increased self-awareness and the ability to express themselves, protest and request inter- *vention. It also discusses how the worker could facilitate them to meet their goals.*

Squires, A. J. (1996) Rehabilitation of Older People, 2nd edn. London: Chapman and Hall.

8 Evaluation of care

Mike Smith

Introduction

This chapter aims to explore the principles relating to evaluation of care. Although many of these principles are common to evaluation generally, reference will be made to specific issues pertinent to rehabilitation nursing. The reasons for evaluation will be outlined providing a basis through which the dimensions and potential methods through which rehabilitation nursing evaluation can be examined.

Evaluation can be defined as:

> 'the critical assessment, on as objective a basis as possible, of the degree to which entire services or their component parts (e.g. diagnostic tests, treatments, caring procedures) fulfil stated goals.'
>
> (St. Leger, Schnieden and Walsworth-Bell, 1993)

Within this definition there are two key principles which are at the basis of evaluation and merit emphasis. Firstly, there is the stated need for objectivity. This is vital should results from evaluation be deemed appropriate, and indicates freedom from any potential bias of the investigators, thus demonstrating the credibility of the information, so enabling use within the clinical setting. Secondly, the reference to fulfilling goals clearly indicates the need to compare against a standard. This could be in the form of a stated aim (e.g. 80% of clients with traumatic brain injury will return to their own home; the client will be able to perform intermittent catheterisation independently) or may be in the form of a comparative standard, such as in a clinical trial setting, whereby the evaluator is aiming to demonstrate an improvement in outcome to that of current interventions (e.g. there will be a 10% reduction in the incidence of bowel accidents if the client performs his bowel programme at the same time on alternate days; a proactive programme of social activities will increase the ability of the individual to engage in conversation with others).

Components of the evaluation process

Due to the often considerable resources required prior to embarking on development of any rehabilitation nursing evaluation process, the key components listed in Box 8.1, adapted from the proposals by the Agency of Health Care Policy and Research (AHCPR, 1992), must be addressed.

Box 8.1
Key components in the evaluation of rehabilitation nursing

- Identification of the persons or agencies requiring the evaluation. Ascertaining why evaluation needs to take place and who are its likely recipients may indicate the content and complexity of the evaluation.
- Identification of which measuring tool(s) are to be used.
- How the evaluation process will be implemented.
- Person(s) responsible for undertaking the evaluation. In the case of issues raised within this chapter, it may be the responsibility of the individual nurse, the rehabilitation nursing team in part or as a whole, or due to the nature of rehabilitation, an interdisciplinary team with rehabilitation nursing as a participating agency.
- Skills required in order to undertake the evaluation effectively. This may indicate training needs needed to undertake the required evaluation.
- The relationships of this information to any other evaluation performed. It is not uncommon for many forms of evaluation to be in use concurrently, particularly in a speciality such as rehabilitation nursing where client problems may be complex. Often valuable additional information can be gained through creating relationships between evaluation tools.

Why evaluate care?

Evaluation of care in rehabilitation nursing is not an optional exercise, it is demanded by all agencies involved in the provision of rehabilitation services (see Figure 8.1).

Clients

Effective evaluation should ensure rehabilitation nursing interventions remain focused on and address the needs and desires of the client and aim towards meaningful client outcomes.

Figure 8.1
Why evaluate care?

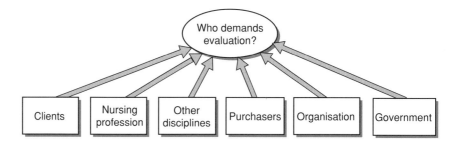

The right of the client to receive care which is demonstrably effective, is indisputable. The voice of clients has been noticeably louder in recent years, reinforced by the Patients Charter. There are ever increasing expectations of health care generally including the field of rehabilitation, with the developments in technology which may impact on the quality of life of these clients. One key point to emphasise is the documented differences between professionals and users of the service in determining how rehabilitation services should be delivered to meet their needs. Although there is now a 'client satisfaction survey' culture developing, it is strongly questionable how comprehensive the majority of these evaluation tools are in guiding and altering rehabilitation practice and services. Most of these tools do not provide sufficient detail to evaluate nursing in rehabilitation. The other related factor which may impact on, and justify the need to evaluate the function and practice of nursing within rehabilitation, is the acceptability to the public of utilising health resources in providing rehabilitation services when compared to other more emotive specialities, e.g. paediatrics. The extent to which this is a problem is unknown, although anecdotally, public opinion appears to favour the latter, which could work against rehabilitation nursing as resources become increasingly limited.

However, currently, public expectations and support of nursing generally appear to be strong, although future developments in the nursing role within health care may influence this either positively or negatively. Public opinion will be further strengthened if nurses can provide evidence of effectiveness through comprehensive evaluation.

Nursing profession

Effective evaluation is at the basis of promoting development of rehabilitation nursing practice for the individual client, clients on a unit, and rehabilitation nursing on a global level. It is at the very foundation of decision-making in the continuous nature of the nursing process.

Evaluation should also aim to indicate the success or otherwise of the processes used to deliver rehabilitation nursing. Not only is it ethically correct to strive for effectiveness and to prove evidence of such within rehabilitation nursing, but evaluation is essential to maintain professional credibility. A lack of such evidence may have perhaps been contributory to the anecdotal belief of the low profile rehabilitation nursing has had in comparison with other rehabilitation disciplines.

Other rehabilitation professionals

There is a necessity for accurate and comprehensive nursing evaluation, as intervention from other team members may often depend on the result of such information. Although this concept is somewhat transferable to other specialities, it is of particular significance in the rehabilitation environment which depends on interdisciplinary teamworking as a fundamental principle of delivering services. It is therefore clear that a major role of the rehabilitation nurse, in providing a unique 24-hour continuum of care, is not only to evaluate prescribed nursing care but also contribute to the evaluation of prescribed interventions of other disciplines.

Purchasers of rehabilitation

The introduction of the white paper 'Working for Patients' (Secretary of State for Health, 1989) has radically altered the health care culture. The resulting purchaser/provider relationship has impacted on rehabilitation units significantly. Despite the apparent bad feeling towards the implications of such a system, purchasers of rehabilitation services do have a right to know that services for which they are paying are effective and efficient. Absence of this evidence may affect the viability of rehabilitation services, as the ability to deliver care in the future is dependent on financial security achieved through continuing purchaser support. The worst scenario is obvious, therefore evaluation of service efficacy is vital to assure rehabilitation services continue to exist for the users of such services.

Organisation

Rehabilitation units rarely exist as independent bodies but are commonly part of larger organisations, often in the form of NHS hospital or community trusts. The organisation as a whole is of course impacted upon through financial security of its services as outlined above. Additionally, a major function of such organisations is to ensure accurate allocation of resources to particular units. A major part of this is the issue of manpower planning. An inability to demonstrate effectiveness and efficiency of the effect of rehabilitation nursing may result in inappropriate skill-mix reviews or inadequate levels of staffing. It seems, anecdotally, that many rehabilitation nursing teams already believe this is happening. It is clear that the only way to halt or reverse this apparent trend is through evaluation, providing evidence of the role of rehabilitation nursing in achievement of positive client outcomes.

Government

Reference to the impact of government legislation has already been described above. Additionally, policies surrounding reducing public sector spending will always affect health. There is a current government-led demand to deliver evidence-based practice. One may suggest that the motive behind this is to enable further cost-cutting to health services generally, and so it may be perceived as threatening to rehabilitation nurses and other professionals. The Department of Health (NHS Executive, 1994) have made reference to evidence-based health care as potentially determining future priorities for funding, stating the intention to:

'Invest an increasing proportion of resources in interventions which are known to be effective and where outcomes can be systematically monitored, and reduce investment in interventions shown to be less effective'.

However, despite concerns regarding the ability of a government to determine correctly what constitutes effectiveness, it surely remains an ethically correct principle to aim to provide evidence that what we do is effective, and therefore we must not lose sight of this fact.

Effectiveness

The reader will already have noted the frequent emphasis on effectiveness. This is a concept worth further exploration as effectiveness can be described using various terms. Five such terms which can relate to effectiveness have been described (St. Leger et al. 1993). These are described below to facilitate clarity.

Efficacy

Efficacy is a term which is used to describe the effect of a particular component part of a service on the individual, e.g. a procedure or intervention, and is based on the principle that this component part must be of benefit if the overall service is to be of benefit, so achieving its overall aims. For example, in the aim of reducing the disability of the individual with paraplegia, if the nurse does not deliver education relating to sexual health, demonstrating efficacy in that particular component of the individual's rehabilitation, the efficacy of the overall aim of reducing disability will be adversely affected.

Efficiency

Efficiency is quite simply concerned with the degree of input required to meet a specific output. It is worth emphasising that, by definition, unless such an output is attained, then a service cannot be described as efficient. An example could be that a client's safe discharge back to their own community is the required output. If the nurse can facilitate this earlier through a new discharge planning scheme on a regular basis, so enabling more clients to utilise a rehabilitation facility throughout a specified period of time, then such a discharge planning scheme would demonstrate a greater efficiency.

Cost-effectiveness

This term relates to the financial costs incurred in meeting a particular outcome. Again, as above, if that outcome is not reached, the term cost-effective is inapplicable. An example of this may be a comparison of the costs and clinical outcome relating to the use of pressure-relieving mattresses against the cost, in terms of time, of more frequent change of position by nursing staff.

This is often a complicated equation. Using the example above, one could question the impact of withdrawing more regular nurse–client contact from a psychological perspective. However, it is uncommon that there is a single nurse intervention on each contact, even if it is just a brief exchange which contributes to a greater understanding of the clients. It is worth noting that the ability to achieve further cost-effectiveness in a service may be impacted upon by the degree of acceptability of the means by which this is to be undertaken. Therefore, although an intervention which may improve cost-effectiveness is identified, it may not be possible to use it unless, both from a client perspective and an ethical viewpoint, such an intervention is deemed acceptable.

Cost-utility

Cost-utility is based on the value which may be given to the outcome of all services. It may be utilised by purchasers in making decisions regarding allocation of resources for alternative services, for example, a head injury service versus a clinic for clients with chronic back pain. Probably the most common tool which could be utilised is that of QALY's (quality adjusted life years), which generate a 'score' relating to quality of life and life-expectancy. When divided by the cost of provision of a service, services can then in theory be compared. This method of allocating resources is fraught with methodological and ethical concerns, which may account for its apparent low usage by purchasers to date.

Cost-benefit

Analysis of cost-benefit usually relates to investigation of similar services, providing a comparison in financial terms of one intervention or service against another in achievement of particular outcomes. It will take into account not only the costs incurred as a result of a particular service, but also the costs related to the impact on society of, for example, the client with a disability, in loss of earnings and need for state benefits. The beneficial effects of the intervention or service will then be measured, again both to society and to the client. An overall cost-benefit can then be determined. As with cost utility, there seems little evidence to date that this process is being utilised frequently in relation to rehabilitation generally or in rehabilitation nursing.

Measurement tools

Prior to exploring specific methods of measurement which may be utilised in evaluation of rehabilitation nursing, from a more general standpoint, it seems worth briefly discussing types of measurement scales and the characteristics thereof.

A measurement tool can be classified as belonging to one of four distinct categories, namely nominal, ordinal, interval or ratio. Although these are often termed 'levels' of measurement, this indicates a form of artificial hierarchy, possibly originating from the scientific world deeming the latter, i.e. ratio scales, as 'purer' in research terms. However, meaningful data can be obtained through the use of any of these 'levels' and therefore the term 'classification' may be more appropriate. Each will be examined in turn, providing an explanation of the classification and related examples in rehabilitation. No attempt will be made to offer an in-depth critical analysis of the classifications, but reference to further reading on this topic is suggested at the end of the chapter.

Nominal measures

Nominal measures are quite simply a method of categorising items into appropriate groups without indicating any particular order. Examples of such measures would include classifying a subject as male or female, English or Scottish, labour or conservative voters, or commonly in health care as a particular diagnosis or impairment, e.g. traumatic brain injury, C6 complete spinal cord injury, Parkinson's disease. Analysis of such measures is restricted to measuring frequencies of subjects assigned to a particular group.

Ordinal measures

Ordinal scales allow the determination of a rank order for a particular set of data, often associated with some form of 'scoring'. It is important to emphasise that a difference in score allows the investigator to make judgements of rank only, and not absolute mathematical accuracy. For example if one was to rank level of pain on a 0–5 scale the difference between a '1' and '2' score would neither indicate the pain was twice as severe, nor indicate an identical difference between a '3' and '4' score.

Their use in rehabilitation seems common in comparison with the other classes of measuring tools. Examples include many of the functional measures related to disability based on an individual's ability to perform certain activities.

Interval measures

The distinct difference between an ordinal and interval scale, as the name suggests, is that an identical interval exists between scores, i.e. the difference between a '2' and '3' is the same as the difference between a '4' and a '5'. An important point to note is that interval measures do not rely on an absolute zero being present in the measuring tool. Probably the most commonly used example in nursing is when measuring temperature, where zero on the Celsius scale would not indicate an absence of temperature, but rather a very low one.

Ratio measures

As with interval measures, the interval between 'scores' is identical, the major difference being the presence of an absolute zero. Examples in practice of ratio measurements would include the timing of a particular activity, for example, walking 10 yards using callipers. Other examples would include weight and height. Clearly there must be an accuracy of the particular measurement used against a gold standard, e.g. the length of a centimetre should be identical no matter which ruler you use.

Figure 8.2
*Characteristics of the
measuring tools*

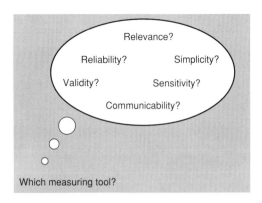

***Characteristics of
measuring tools***

Key to the process of evaluation or measurement is determining whether the measuring tool is appropriate to the relevant situation. Wade (1992) suggested six factors which require consideration prior to choosing a measuring tool. These are illustrated in Figure 8.2 and briefly discussed below.

Relevance

The effort required in the collection of data is expensive in resource terms, not only from a financial perspective, but, particularly pertinent in today's climate, the rehabilitation nurse's most precious asset, i.e. time. It is essential that the measure is specific to the individual needs of a particular situation, ensuring not only that enough data is collected but equally important, that not too much data is collected for the particular task.

Validity

In terms of measurement, a valid tool can be defined as one which measures what it is designed to measure. Many types of validity have been described, which other texts cover in great detail and will therefore not be addressed within this chapter. Suffice to say that there are many aspects to validity, e.g. environmental, the potential presence of other impairments, time-scale (particularly in retrospective studies) and ability to predict outcome.

Reliability

Reliability relates to the repeatability of the observation, and may be described in terms of the same score being obtained by the same observer, or the same score being obtained by two or more different observers. Statistical measures do exist which aim to measure the reliability of a particular measure, and which should be used as appropriate. Influencing factors on reliability include the provision of adequate training for observers and the complexity of the measure being used.

Sensitivity

Sensitivity relates to the ability of the tool to detect change. In simple terms for example, an ordinal scale which offers three alternatives would not be as sensitive as one which offered ten points when measuring the same variable. Consequently, a scale which is not sensitive enough may not produce meaningful results, whereas a scale which is too complex in nature may affect reliability due to recording error.

Simplicity   Related to sensitivity, simplicity refers to the user-friendliness of the measurement. A tool which is simple in design and requires clear and concise responses will both aid compliance, particularly when completed by a client, and positively affect the reliability of the observation.

Communicability   This refers to the ease with which the results can be reported and understood by others. This is an essential component if the results of any measurement are designed to affect the practice of rehabilitation nursing outside the practice of the investigator themselves.

The development of new measuring tools is far from being a quick and easy task if one is to ensure that all the above characteristics are present. Therefore, the author would strongly condone the approach taken by Wade (1990), who advocated investigating the potential use of existing measures and assessing their suitability to the task, prior to development of a new measurement tool.

Methods of evaluating care

The examples, definitions and descriptions given earlier stress that the concept of effectiveness of care is based on the aim of meeting goals or standards, which therefore suggests that evaluation of effectiveness is focused on achievement, or otherwise, of outcome. The principles of structure (essentially represented by a service's fixed costs), process (how the service is organised) and outcome (the impact or result of a service) originating from the work of Donabedian (1980), have been enthusiastically grasped not only by nursing, but commonly throughout all aspects of health care provision. Indeed, it is often such a framework which has been the basis for the development of standards in nursing. Despite an acceptance of the importance in measuring all of these dimensions as methods of evaluation, the author would wish to offer a cautionary note. The fact that the terms structure, process and outcome are all written and expressed in that particular order should not be perceived as the order in which the development of services should be viewed, even if this reflects what may have happened in reality. Surely the first stage in any service development or evaluation should be against the aim or goal of the service, i.e. the outcome, which should then determine the optimum process to achieve this, which in turn should indicate the required resources or structure. The question could therefore be raised as to whether these principles should be expressed and termed outcome, process, structure. Although this may appear slightly pedantic, the philosophical importance of this in the development and evaluation of rehabilitation nursing would not only ensure they are viewed in the correct

Figure 8.3
Dimensions in the evaluation of care in rehabilitation nursing

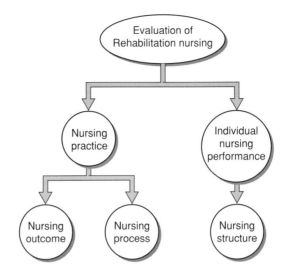

order, but would promote this way of thinking to more junior colleagues whose understanding may not be as great. One could argue that evaluating rehabilitation nursing practice cuts across the dimensions of outcome and process, whereas evaluation of nursing performance (the degree and scope of skills required in order to practice) sits more comfortably within the dimension of structure. These distinct dimension of evaluation for rehabilitation nursing are illustrated in Figure 8.3. Although obviously closely interrelated, for the purpose of explanation each will be described in turn, outlining the content of the evaluation. Additionally, potentially appropriate methods which may be undertaken in each dimension will be suggested.

Evaluation of nursing outcomes

Evaluation is integral in the 'nursing process' and is continuous in nature, involving both the nurse and the client. It should enable determination of client progress against set goals formulated at the planning stage, with either the nurse exclusively, or (more commonly in rehabilitation) through collaboration and in consultation with the interdisciplinary team. It enables planned interventions to be maintained as currently prescribed, modified, reprioritised or even abandoned, if the intervention is evaluated to be ineffective.

Evaluation in nursing practice may occur on a continual basis as care is being delivered, i.e. formatively. Alternatively, evaluation may compare progress against the set goals on a 'snap-shot' basis, usually related to documentation of care at the end of shift, i.e. summatively. The latter may also be termed 'concurrent outcome'.

While analysing the results of the evaluation, one of four potential scenarios exist. These are:

- the expected result has not been achieved
- some aspects of the objectives have been achieved

- new or different priorities have been identified
- the goal has been achieved

If progress towards meeting client goals related to nursing activity has not been entirely achieved, the evaluating nurse must question the reason for this. It may be that goals set were unrealistic in time or resources, or the client did not want to or did not have the capability to meet the goal. The care plan must also be examined to ensure full implementation, from both the nursing and client perspective. As a result of answers to these questions, a need to modify the care plan as appropriate may arise.

The term clinical indicator is a measurement which may indicate acceptable performance or otherwise of health care professionals. Two categories of clinical indicator exist, that of rate-based and sentinel event. A rate-based indicator specifies a level by which a regularly occurring outcome is below or above an acceptable level, e.g. 30% of patients on intermittent catheterisation will have asymptomatic bacteriuria. A sentinel event will investigate on an individual basis a rarely occurring incident, for example, a patient sustaining serious injury as a result of a fall out of bed. It is the former of these two which is commonly related to measurement of outcome.

Measurement of clinical outcome is concerned with the impact of health services on individuals and communities, and appears to be gaining momentum amongst purchasers and providers of rehabilitation as a worthwhile, indeed vital, exercise to undertake. Providers of rehabilitation can potentially use outcome measures, firstly, to enable most efficient utilisation of all internal resources, including personnel and financial. Secondly, it can be a baseline by which the success or otherwise of alternate interventions or processes can be ascertained. In principle, these should be interdisciplinary measures of outcome (Freeman, Hobart and Thompson, 1996), however, nursing as a profession must develop systems whereby the nursing contribution to outcome can be extracted both in practice and process. This is the only obviously effective means by which we can evaluate our own performance and so validate and justify nursing within rehabilitation. This is also where we can impact most, as our ability and influence to change rehabilitation is strongest in changing our own contribution, rather than attempting to change the contributions made by other professions. In view of this need for working towards positive interdisciplinary outcomes, one could strongly suggest that the aim of rehabilitation nursing should mirror the aim of rehabilitation generally, which has been proposed as 'the reduction of disability and handicap'. Additionally, in view of the need to prevent secondary complications, not uncommon in clients with complex disability, one could also logically propose that rehabilitation should aim to minimise the incidence of related potential impairments, e.g.

pressure sores and contractures of limbs. The classifications of impairment, disability and handicap proposed by the WHO (1980) have been suggested by some authors as potential variables through which rehabilitation outcomes can be measured. Quality of life measures have also been suggested as a potentially worthwhile additional measure of outcome. Despite the potential benefit of measuring impairment in some specific instances, the author will focus on the other three measures in discussing nursing contribution to outcome, i.e. disability, handicap and quality of life.

Disability Disability has been defined as a restriction or lack of ability to perform an activity in the manner considered normal for a human being (WHO, 1980). Disturbance of function involves, for example, a reduced ability to communicate, walk or dress. Commonly utilised disability measures include the functional independence measure (FIM) (Hamilton et al. 1987), and the Barthel index (Mahoney and Barthel 1965).

Handicap Handicap has been defined as:

> *'A disadvantage for a given individual resulting from an impairment or a disability that limits or prevents the fulfilment of a role that is normal (depending on age, sex, social and cultural factors) for that individual'.*

> (WHO, 1980)

Figure 8.4 illustrates the six dimensions of societal function.

Although there is obviously a significant proportion of handicap which is as a result of societal influences, a feeling commonly expressed by some authors who have a disability themselves, entering into this topic more fully is not within the remit of this chapter. However, the strength of societal influences would suggest the wisdom of moving the emphasis away from the hospital-based rehabilitation programme, which appears often impairment- and

Figure 8.4
Dimensions of societal function

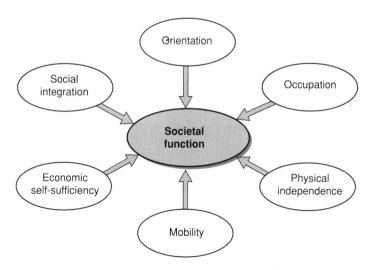

disability-focused (following either a 'medical' or therapy-type 'functional' model), to community living of the individual who requires rehabilitation services. If one is to accept this basic philosophy, questions must be raised about the current location of rehabilitation resources and services. However, such issues are covered in detail in other chapters and evaluation of the nursing contribution in a particular rehabilitation environment, in reducing handicap as an outcome, is what is being discussed here.

Commonly used measures of handicap include the Craig Handicap Assessment and Recording Technique or 'CHART' (Whiteneck et al., 1990) and the Environmental Status Scale (International Federation of Multiple Sclerosis Societies, 1985).

Quality of life

Despite the nursing and rehabilitation literature containing many references to quality of life, there seems to be a lack of a common definition, and therefore clarity, as to what constitutes this most commonly utilised term (Ferrans and Powers, 1985). Most have reference to a perception of some value or excellence in aspects of life (Ware and Sherbourne, 1992). There is usually a degree of comparison which may indicate either a good or poor quality of life, and the term is frequently used in an evaluative manner (Meeberg, 1993). The majority of measurement tools are multidimensional in nature and contain subjective (the client's satisfaction with a situation) and possibly objective components (a societal value of the situation, e.g. living conditions). Once again, the author would urge the reader, in consideration of an appropriate tool, to adhere to the principles outlined above and refer to further texts.

Evaluation of nursing processes

Since processes can be defined as the way in which the service is organised and performed, such processes have a direct bearing on the effectiveness of service delivery. Despite the importance of ascertaining the success or otherwise of the various processes utilised, they can often be difficult to measure, and occasionally to directly influence, due to the involvement and interaction of the many agencies involved in health care. This is particularly pertinent in the field of rehabilitation of those individuals with a complex disability, where the intervention of a team of professionals is commonly recognised as the best approach to utilise. However, one could hypothesise that the established close and often interdisciplinary approach which rehabilitation has embraced would contribute well to evaluation of process, when compared to health care situations where such teamworking is not so integral and where such co-operation between agencies is not commonplace.

Rehabilitation nursing philosophies of care

Such philosophies are statements which not only indicate beliefs about rehabilitation nursing practice and process but additionally can be utilised both to guide nursing developments and essentially promote a common clear vision for the entire nursing team. Philosophies, however, should not be set in stone indefinitely but should be dynamic documents enabling these beliefs to be updated as changes occur in health care, and in the expectations of clients, and nursing staff generally.

Quality   The WHO (1989) stated that under the umbrella of quality assurance programmes, four components required consideration:

- client satisfaction with provided services
- professional performance, i.e. technical ability
- Resource use, i.e. efficiency
- Risk management, i.e. the risk of illness or injury associated with the service.

Six key elements of quality have been defined (Maxwell, 1984) and are illustrated in Figure 8.5. As the issues relating to the elements of effectiveness and efficiency have been covered earlier, for each of the remaining elements, a definition will be indicated and an example from rehabilitation nursing offered.

Appropriateness relates to the relevance of the service to the needs of the client. An example of inappropriateness in rehabilitation nursing would be the involvement of the client in recreational activities which they have no interest or desire to continue after rehabilitation is completed. A recent client indicated that he had spent years 'bunking off' games sessions at school only to be instructed to participate in sports activities during his inpatient hospital rehabilitation programme.

Equity indicates the need to provide equal services for all. For example, every client should have the opportunity to have access to a formal client educational programme or appropriate support from community rehabilitation nurses.

Figure 8.5
Elements of quality

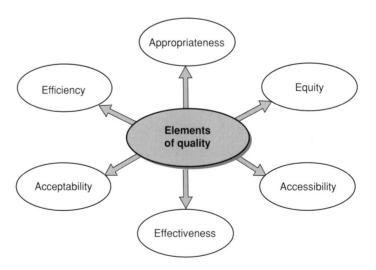

Accessibility is defined as the ease with which services are obtainable. This may encompass limitations in mobility capability, waiting times and knowledge that services exist. A recent small-scale focus group study undertaken at the London Spinal Injuries Unit in Stanmore (Smith, 1996) highlighted that, for persons with spinal cord injury, the inability to access information on a regular basis was a major problem when living in the community with a disability. Examples related to this could include ensuring that a client is aware of appropriate support groups within his local area, or of accurate information relating to recent developments which may impact positively on their level of disability.

Acceptability focuses on the degree to which reasonable expectations of the client are satisfied. A question must be raised as to whether we actually know what client expectations of rehabilitation, and in particular, rehabilitation nursing, actually are. To some degree acceptability should be achieved if rehabilitation teams are employing a truly client-focused service.

The principle of total quality management is based on involvement of all members of an organisation and expands across discipline and professional boundaries, it is a continuous dynamic process. A clinical and managerial framework that commits staff to producing a systematic continuous process of evaluating agreed levels of care and service provision should be provided. Although quality appears to be viewed as an additional extra, on top of existing workload, it should be in essence, an integral part of providing rehabilitation nursing services.

Nursing audit

By definition, nursing audit is a quality assurance mechanism for monitoring and evaluating the quality of interventions provided by nursing. The audit process has distinct stages which can be used to evaluate any practice within the rehabilitation setting, as outlined in Box 8.2.

Box 8.2
The stages of the adit process

1. Identification of the practice or intervention to be evaluated.
2. Development of standard which the audit team believe is acceptable.
3. Development of criteria necessary to achieve the standard often written using the terms structure, process, outcome.
4. Steps 1 and 2 form the basis of the audit tool.
5. The auditor(s) are trained in the use of the tool to maximise reliability.
6. The auditors perform the audit utilising the criteria and 'rules' for assessment.
7. Results from the audit are analysed indicating 'problem areas'.
8. Development of an action plan using a standard objective setting format with the rehabilitation team.

> 9. A date for reaudit is agreed.
>
> Stages 4 to 9 may be described as the 'audit cycle'.

Audit versus research

Although discussing research in rehabilitation nursing is not within the remit of this chapter, as there, anecdotally, appears to be a degree of confusion amongst clinical nursing staff regarding audit and research, it is worthwhile to outline both the similarities and the definite differences between the two (see Table 8.1).

Integrated care pathways

Originating in the USA and commonly from acute services, 'clinical care pathways' or 'integrated care pathways' are a tool which can serve both as a guide to processes involved in rehabilitation, and also an audit tool giving guidance as to improvements which can be made to a service. They appear to be commonplace in the USA, where there role is undoubtedly partly financial, reflecting the nature of health care on the other side of the Atlantic. It is probably for this reason that their implementation in this country has been somewhat slower in comparison, and although some evidence does now exist in a few practice areas, there appears to be little in the nursing literature to date which indicates their usefulness or otherwise in the UK

Hotchkiss (1997) identified six main features of an integrated pathway system.

- It is the sole multidisciplinary plan and record of client care.
- It is commonly located near or with the client and is paper-based. It is probable, however, with the increased utilisation of information technology within health care, that this will become computerised on a network system, to allow individual team members to input data in their own department. Additionally, a benefit of this may be in the speed by which this information can be analysed.
- It provides information relating not only to the intervention to be carried out but also the sequence, timescale and person or discipline responsible. It is therefore fairly simplistic to extract the nursing intervention and evaluate if and when such an intervention occurred.
- Variances from the plan are recorded and analysed. Baldry and Rossiter (1995), in outlining the implementation of an integrated care pathway to a UK neuro-rehabilitation unit, described the use of a variance sheet utilised when either the intervention was not implemented or the specific goal not reached. Included on such a sheet must be the reason for the variance. Potential variance codes were outlined in a preliminary study undertaken within the same unit (Rossiter and Thompson, 1995), under the categories of client/family/carers, clinician, external system (e.g. community care issues) and internal system (e.g. problems relating to

Table 8.1
Similarities and differences between audit and research

	Audit	Research
Purpose	Monitor and improve practice at a local level	Provision of additional scientific knowledge to base clinical practice upon
Process	Analysis of quality Cyclical process affecting local practice	Scientific enquiry Linear process contributing to knowledge which can be generalised to populations or clinical groups
Basis	Driven by local needs or problems	Driven by existing knowledge and theory
Methods	Utilises data which exists as a result of current clinical practice	Utilises data which often requires the use of additional measuring tools
Sample	Local clinical significance is required. May be obtained through measurement agaisnt a standard with one or more clients	Statistical significance is required to produce results which can be generalised. Strict inclusion criteria are necessary and often large groups of clients
Reporting of findings	Primarily those local staff working in the environment which has been audited. Standard and audit tool may merit dissemination to other similar centres	Responsibility to disseminate results widely due to the ability to use the results on a global scale
Timescale	Changes in practice are immediate and ongoing as part of the audit cycle	Changes in practice may take a significant period of time

availability of department or equipment). These categories are almost identical to those described in the work of Hotchkiss (1997), whose main amendment was the discrete separation of nurse omission from that of the clinician. From a rehabilitation nursing point of view, this would make analysis easier, and therefore seems to be a reasonable step to take. However, at the risk of nurses feeling as though they have been somehow singled out for scrutiny, the author would suggest a further positive development may be to do likewise, for all the core disciplines involved in rehabilitation.

- A plan or practice may be adjusted following audit of the variances.
- Due to the pre-printed nature of integrated care pathways, there is minimal freetext.

There are concerns raised anecdotally regarding the use of integrated pathways. However, these do not appear to be reflected in practice from the literature to date from those authors who have described their use. Conversely, feedback has been almost entirely positive in nature (Metcalf, 1991; Rossiter and Thompson, 1995). Notably, improvements in cross-discipline communication, a reduction in duplication of information within documentation, and facilitation of staff training and orientation/induction programmes have been documented. Additionally, and most importantly, pathways evaluate and, through the audit process, impact positively on the care provision, process and outcome. Although this author is indeed enthusiastic regarding the use of integrated care pathways, it is clear that much further work is needed to determine if such benefits as described above are actually commonplace, and to convince others in rehabilitation that development of these is worthwhile.

Evaluation of nursing structure

The context for the work of a service is largely set by the 'structure'. It seems common sense to state that the environment in which rehabilitation nursing is taking place should facilitate rather than inhibit the process. This incorporates the relatively stable characteristics of the service, such as the distribution and qualifications of the personnel, and the way in which the staff are structured. As rehabilitation nursing skills and experience are required as part of the resources, within this section the evaluation and development of the individual nurse will be explored. Other aspects of structure include the actual physical environment and available equipment, which will also be addressed.

The success of nursing interventions, measured through the influence on promoting effective client outcome, is dependent on the performance of individual nurses. Evaluation of nurse performance in care delivery is vital to develop strategies which truly impact on development in providing effective care for both the current individual client and others in the future. Three techniques for development of the individual nurse will be explored: reflective practice, individual performance review or appraisal, and peer assessment.

Figure 8.6
The reflective process

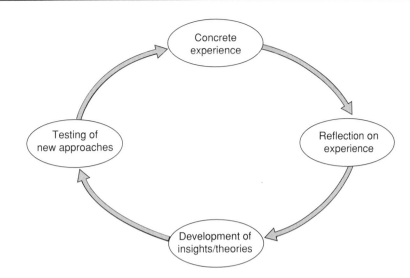

Reflective practice

It was the publication of *The Reflective Practitioner: How Professionals Think in Action* (Schon 1983) which opened the way for a distinct role for reflective practice in nursing. There now seems to be widespread acceptance in the UK of this technique and it is perceived as essential for professional development. Similarities with experiential learning models are obvious and form the basis for effective development of the individual nurse, facilitating ever-improving competence in delivery of care. Such a process is cyclical in nature and can be illustrated as in Figure 8.6.

A concrete practical nursing intervention or experience which the nurse considers problematic, or of interest, forms the topic for reflection. The experience is evaluated, gathering observations and information, and is reflected upon. This analysis of the experience results in the nurse developing certain insights and theories of how the experience could be improved upon. These insights and theories can then be utilised to generate new practical approaches to similar interventions or experiences in the future. The use of journals and diaries have been described to formalise this form of evaluation, particularly within the context of nurse education.

One criticism that the author would make of current work on reflection is that it appears to be written in language that most junior rehabilitation nurses would find at best heavy reading, rather than offering concise practical guidance on the actual process of reflection. To this end, Box 8.3 attempts to offer a concise guide in a checklist format which may assist the rehabilitation nurse at any level to reflect on practice.

Box 8.3
Reflection – A practical Checklist

1. Write a description of the experience and highlight the key issues which merit attention.
2. Reflect on:

> The aim of the intervention
> Results of the intervention on the client
> Implications of the intervention on self and other staff members
> How you felt during the experience.
> 3. What factors both from previous experience and previous knowledge influenced your actions?
> 4. What experiences and knowledge which you did not possess prior to the event would have helped your decision-making?
> 5. What alternative choices could have been utilised and what may have been the result?
> 6. What learning has taken place, examining:
> How this experience has increased personal knowledge and will change practice in the future when faced with similar events.
> How you feel now about the event and what support is available to assist in dealing with those feelings.
> Should this learning be shared with others to add to their knowledge?

It is worth pointing out that this is not a technique which has received total support in the literature. Limitations outlined include the fallibility of recall (Newell, 1992) and therefore its effect on accurate reflection. Also, a phenomenon termed 'hindsight bias' has been described, whereby the practitioner's knowledge of utilised interventions and actual outcome may influence accurate objective reflection on events, as opposed to interpretation by someone viewing the situation totally independently (Jones, 1995). However, this author would wish to emphasise that these views, however valid, should not detract from the positive aspects of reflection, with the ultimate aim of development of the individual nurse.

Individual performance review

Performance review is a two-way process between manager and post-holder designed to provide a framework for development of the individual nurse. It is based on appraisal of the nurse in delivering care and the need for self-development. There are obvious similarities between this and the development of learning contracts used in the spheres of pre-registration and post-registration nurse education. It consists of the components illustrated in Figure 8.7.

Areas for development are identified from a practical perspective, emphasising the usefulness of both individual self-appraisal through reflection as discussed above, and also peer assessment. It should, however, be a tool focused, not only on areas for development, but should also encourage the optimum use of individual perceived strengths, so contributing to the development of the ward nursing team generally. For example, should a nurse possess practical experience of performing audit above that of colleagues, it would be

Figure 8.7
*Individual perfor-
mance review*

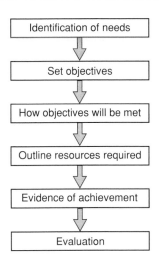

Identification of needs

Set objectives

How objectives will be met

Outline resources required

Evidence of achievement

Evaluation

wasteful not to incorporate use of this within an individual performance review. We are very good at focusing on weaknesses to the
detriment of providing opportunities to utilise strengths. Of course
weaknesses must be managed, however there must be an acceptance that the unique variety of experiences and positive strengths
which different members of the rehabilitation nursing team may
have, contribute to the overall functioning of the team. This is congruent with recognised authors describing effective teamworking
(Belbin, 1994) and despite the emphasis on teamworking in the
environment in which we work, rehabilitation nursing does not
seem to be exempt from this wasteful approach. The contractual
nature of the individual performance review process indicates the
responsibility of the manager to provide the necessary resources,
both financial and educational, to enable objectives to be met.

Peer review   Peer review has been described as:

> '*A critical evaluation of one's clinical practice by colleagues
> who are equal in education, qualifications or position and are
> therefore able to make qualitative judgements concerning clin-
> ical performance.*'

(Leibold 1983)

It seems to have originated in the USA in the early 1970s. If this
is a concept which is to be employed, it is the responsibility of
rehabilitation nurse managers to encourage the development of an
environment which facilitates this. It is a process which must be
accepted by all participants before implementation. Creating acceptance of a technique which is certainly alien to most UK rehabilitation nurses may take a significant amount of persuasion, education
and support. The author would suggest that achieving the level of
trust necessary to give the average UK rehabilitation nurse the ability to pass judgement on a colleague may be the greatest challenge.

However, practical approaches to implement peer review which may be less direct and therefore perceived as 'safer' could include the nurse presenting a case study or critical incident in which he or she may have had involvement and, using the principles of reflective practice as outlined later in this chapter, the relevant peer(s) could offer suggestion as to how intervention could have been improved. If no such event is obvious, particular scenarios could be created. It does seem philosophically sound to promote this concept rather than the top-down methods of appraisal often employed. This would certainly reinforce the principle that quality of performance is the responsibility of the practitioners, as opposed to a responsibility solely of management, and so assist the rehabilitation nursing team to view quality as an integral part of their role, rather than an additional extra on top of other responsibilities.

This could also be extended to look at group performance. It is often within a group setting that standards will be determined or goals set and appraisal of potential options to solving a particular problem occur. Obvious benefits of this approach are that of gaining different viewpoints on the aspects of service delivery and encouraging nursing team acceptance due to increased ownership of the solution. This now occurs in some centres, with all the rehabilitation team members present to some degree within the process of goal planning (Kennedy, 1991). However, the author is unaware of centres that have formally utilised this process to evaluate purely rehabilitation nursing.

Evaluation of the rehabilitation environment

There is little solid evidence of appropriate tools which would facilitate evaluation of the environment in which rehabilitation nursing is to take place, and indeed the possible impact of environmental differences on outcome. These could be divided into issues for the client (Box 8.4) and issues for nursing (Box 8.5) (although some may be issues for both parties), and the author would suggest these issues as potential areas for investigation of a hospital rehabilitation environment. These are not designed to be exhaustive lists, but are provided to stimulate the reader into thinking about suitable aspects for their own working environment.

Box 8.4
Client issues concerning the rehabilitation environment

1. Client access to areas within the rehabilitation environment with the aim of optimising rather than limiting independence. This would include the broader aspects of minimising the impact of the relevant disability, e.g. clear signs suitable for clients with visual impairments.
2. Floor coverings.
3. Temperature of the environment.
4. Availability of recreational/relaxation facilities.
5. Access to areas which allow privacy.

Box 8.5
Nursing issues concerning the rehabilitation environment

1. The physical space available to perform interventions
2. Areas for meetings and educational activities
3. Sufficient storage space
4. Sufficient manual handling aids and other general health and safety assistive devices.
5. If computerised systems are to be used, sufficient terminals and keyboards
6. Easy access to other rehabilitation team members
7. Appropriate client to nurse, and nurse to nurse communication systems
8. Appropriate systems and facilities for the safe disposal of clinical waste and general rubbish
9. Support from domestic, portering and cleaning services within the rehabilitation area
10. Sufficient supplies

Nursing skill-mix in rehabilitation

Clearly, assessment of both appropriate nursing staffing numbers and relevant grades and experience is not possible to undertake accurately and effectively unless the contribution of nursing within rehabilitation is clear. One common attempt to evaluate the need for nursing staffing levels has been the emergence of the client dependency score. Through determining the numbers of nurses required for varying dependency and measuring the dependency of clients in a particular service, alterations could be made to those staffing levels as dependency changes. Although in principle this appears logical, unless there is a degree of constant flexibility in the manner by which duty rosters are set, this may only be useful in establishment changes year on year. This appears far from satisfactory. Simple dependency scores do not indicate levels of experience or skill-mix required. More complex tools may allow this to a degree. Such a tool, which allocates a particular score to each specific nurse intervention, may provide useful information towards the undertaking of this task through relating each intervention to a grade of nurse. Additionally, through the totalling of scores, an overall dependency score for each and all of the clients could be ascertained.

Communicating evaluation

One final point which must be emphasised is the issue of communication of nursing evaluation. Channels of communication must be not only identified but utilised. Traditionally in the UK, nurses have seemed quiet compared to other disciplines in relating the value of their role and contributions to health care to others. A prime example of this is in rehabilitation nursing. One need look no further than the low profile nursing has, not only outside nursing, but also inside the profession itself in comparison with our therapy and medical colleagues. Publication of rehabilitation nursing-led initiatives, opinions and research in the UK has been sparse at best, and although in no way advocating a US-style health care system, it is indisputable that we could learn from our rehabilitation nursing colleagues on the other side of the Atlantic, who seem to be able to undertake this with remarkable fluency in comparison.

Rehabilitation nurses in the UK must start to 'shout from the rooftops', we must let all who demand evidence of effectiveness in health care as outlined above, recognise how valuable the contribution of nursing is through the results of our evaluation.

Conclusion   Despite the lip-service often paid to the importance of evaluation in practice, with the exception of the evaluation performed as part of the day-to-day nursing process, other forms of evaluation have appeared to be less popular in the past. However, the increased demand on health care resources have somewhat twisted the arms of rehabilitation services to view these other methods of evaluation as essential to the continuation of these services, as well as a desire to improve rehabilitation practice through development. The ever-increasing demands upon the time available for 'practical hands-on nursing' of 'add-ons' such as clinical audit, seem commonly verbalised by today's rehabilitation nurse. It is, however, not only vital that this attitude is challenged and corrected but it is demanded by those who we serve. The only remedy to this is a cultural change which recognises, in the form of action, both theoretically and more importantly practically, that evaluation is an integral part of rehabilitation nursing, not only for the benefit of the client but also for the development, and possibly the very survival, of rehabilitation nursing.

Questions for discussion

- Can we objectively measure all the aspects of the role and contributions of the rehabilitation nurse?
- Look at your own practice area, to what extent is the nursing practice objectively evaluated?
- Have rehabilitation nurses got the skills to effectively evaluate their practice?
- What are the major barriers to the rehabilitation nurse's ability to evaluate?
- Is effective evaluation the means by which rehabilitation nursing can gain a higher profile within rehabilitation in the UK?

References
Agency for Health Care Policy and Research (AHCPR) (1992). *Using Clinical Practice Guidelines to Evaluate Quality of Care.* Rockville MD: US Department of Health and Human resource services.

Baldry, J.A. & Rossiter, D. (1995) Introduction of integrated care pathways to a neurorehabilitation unit. *Physiotherapy*, **81**.
Belbin, M. (1994) *Team Roles at Work.* Oxford: Butterworth Heinemann.

Donabedian, A. (1980) *Explorations in Quality Assessment and Monitoring Vol. 1: The definition of quality and approaches to its assessment*. Ann Arbour: Health Administration Press.

Ferrans, C.E. Powers, M.J. (1985) Quality of life index: development and pyschometric properties. *Advances in Nursing Science*, **8**, 15–24.

Freeman, J.A., Hobart, J.C. & Thompson, A.J. (1996) Outcomes-based research in neuro-rehabilitation: the need for multidisciplinary team involvement. *Disability and Rehabilitation*, **18**, 106–110.

Hamilton, B., Granger, C.V., Sherwin, F.S., Zielezny, M. & Tashman, T. S. (1987) A uniform national data system for medical rehabilitation. In *Rehabilitation Outcomes Analysis and Measurement*, ed. Fuhrer, M.J. Baltimore: Brooks.

Hotchkiss, R. (1997) Integrated care pathways. *NTResearch*, **2**, 30–37.

International Federation of Multiple Sclerosis Societies (1985) *Minimal Record of Disability*. New York: National Multiple Sclerosis Society.

Jones, P.R. (1995) Hindsight bias in reflective practice: An empirical investigation. *Journal of Advanced Nursing*, **21**, 783–785.

Kennedy, P., Walker, L. & White, D. (1991) Ecological evaluation of goal planning and advocacy in a rehabilitation enviroment for spinal cord injured people. *Paraplegia*, **29**, 197–202.

McGrath, J.R. & Davies, A.M. (1992) Rehabilitation – where do we go and how do we get there. *Clinical Rehabilitation*, **6**, 225–235.

Metcalf, E.M. (1991) The orthopaedic critical path. *Orthopaedic Nursing*, **10**, 25–31.

Mahoney, F. & Barthel, D.W. (1965) Functional evaluation – the Barthel index. *MD State Medical Journal*, **14**, 342–346.

Maxwell, R.J. (1984) Quality assessment in health. *British Medical Journal*, **288**, 1470–1471.

Meeberg, G.A. (1993) Quality of life: a concept analysis. *Journal of Advanced Nursing*, **18**, 32–38.

Newell, R. (1992) Reflection: art, science or pseudoscience. *Nurse Education Today*, **14**, 79–81.

NHS Executive (1994) *Priorities and Planning Guidance for the NHS 1995/96*, (EL (94) 55). NHS Executive. Leeds:

Rossiter, D. & Thompson, A.J. (1995) Introduction of integrated pathways for patients with multiple sclerosis in an inpatient neurorehabilitation setting. *Disability and Rehabilitation*, **17**, 443–448.

St Leger, A.S., Schnieden, H. & Walsworth-Bell, J.P. (1993). *Evaluating Health Services' Effectiveness*. Milton Keyness: Open University Press.

Schon (1983). *The Reflective Practitioner: How Professionals Think in Action*. London: Temple Smith.

Secretary of State for Health (1989) *Working for Patients*. London: HMSO.

Smith, M.J. (1996) Expectations of rehabilitation – a focus group project (unpublished). Paper presented at the American Association of SCI nurses. Las Vegas; September 1997.

Wade, D.T. (1992) Measurement in neurological rehabilitation. Oxford: Oxford University Press.

Ware, J. E. & Sherbourne, C. D. (1992) A 36 item short-form survey (SF-36). *Medical Care*, **30**, 473–483.

Whiteneck, G., Charlifue, S., Gerhart, K., Overholser, J. & Richardson, G. (1992) Quantifying handicap, a new measure of long term outcomes. *Archives of Physical and Medical Rehabilitation*, **73**, 519–526.

World Health Organisation (1980) *International Classification of Impairments, Disabilities and Handicaps*. Geneva: WHO.

World Health Organisation (1989) *Quality Assurance in Health Care*, Vol 1, No. 2/3. Geneva: WHO.

Further reading

Parsley, K. & Corrigan, P. (1994) *Quality Improvement in Nursing and Healthcare*. London: Chapman and Hall.

Pilling, D. & Watson, G. (1995) *Evaluating Quality in Services for Disabled and Older People*. London: Jessica Knigsley Publishing.

St Leger, A. S., Schnieden, H. & Walsworth-Bell, J.P. (1993). *Evaluating Health Services' Effectiveness*. Milton Keynes: Open University Press.

Wade, D.T. (1990) *Measurement in Neurological Rehabilitation*. Oxford: Oxford University Press.

SECTION

3 ISSUES IN REHABILITATION NURSING

9 The relationship health promotion a rehabilitation

Sally Davis

Key issues
- Health promotion
- Health education
- Health promotion and rehabilitation
- Nurse's role in health promotion
- Health promotion model for rehabilitation nurses

Introduction

This chapter will explore the relationship between health promotion and rehabilitation and will put forward the view that if rehabilitation is viewed as health promotion, then nurses and other professionals would focus more clearly on wellness rather than illness.

Rehabilitation is generally described in the literature as maximising the physical, psychological, social, economic, vocational and educational status of an individual (Henderson and Nite, 1978; Melvin, 1989; Teague, Cipriano and McGhee, 1990). However, according to Melvin (1989) this approach does not provide an effective framework on which to organise treatment strategies. Wade (1996) advocates the use of the WHO (1980) ICIDH model which describes pathology, impairment, disability and handicap. This model allows for the following definition of rehabilitation:

> *'Rehabilitation is a re-iterative, problem solving, educational process focusing on disability and aiming to reduce handicap, client and family distress, all within the limitations imposed by the pathology and resources available.'*
>
> (Wade, 1996)

Enabling individuals to resume roles lost, which is at the level of handicap, can be identified as being the ultimate goal of rehabilitation (Melvin, 1989; Wade, 1990). Professionals working in rehabilitation have generally viewed disability as a stable entity, with the emphasis being on the client's recovery of their former self, rather than on disability as a condition that is undergoing change all the time (Brandon, 1985; Marge, 1988). This has resulted in rehabilitation services being developed in the areas of intervention strategies,

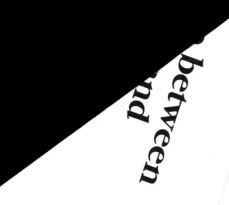

l coordination of services, but not incorporating health
programmes (Teague et al., 1990). The absence of
motion programmes in rehabilitation could account for
being viewed as stable. The incorporation of health pro-
programmes would focus on disability as undergoing
Health promotion can be identified as having more of a
and change potential than rehabilitation (Brandon, 1985).
could argue, therefore, that rehabilitation is health promotion,
the same goals.

proi..

ue to its different interpretations, health promotion is a difficult
concept to define, which could account for it not being utilised to its
full potential within rehabilitation. The Ottawa Charter for Health
Promotion (WHO, 1986) describes it as a process which enables people to increase control over their health and improve it.
Rehabilitation needs to be the same active process if individuals are
to resume specific roles: the goal of rehabilitation. The WHO (1986)
definition equates with the previously stated view of disability as
being a condition that is undergoing change all the time (Brandon,
1985; Marge, 1988). Tannahill (1985) suggests that, although the
philosophy underlying the WHO (1986) definition is sound, it is too
vague for practical purposes. The overall goal of health promotion
can be identified as being to increase the physical, mental and social
facets of positive health in a balanced way, and also to prevent physical, mental and social ill-health (Downie, Fyfe and Tannahill, 1990).

Pender (1987) describes it as being an activity that is concerned
with sustaining or increasing one's level of wellbeing, self actualisa-
tion and personal fulfillment. Wellbeing and personal fulfillment are
subjective concepts. What may be a high level of wellbeing for one
person may not be for another. According to Nutbeam (1986), in
health promotion, the term 'wellbeing' might focus more on social
integration and support, placing it within the social model of health.
It could be said that wellbeing is to do with how one is feeling and
is generally equated to a high self esteem. Clients going through the
rehabilitation process generally have a low self esteem. They have
lost control over their lives, and are experiencing constant change.
Rehabilitation should therefore be aiming to increase their level of
control, and ultimately their level of wellbeing.

The definitions of health promotion discussed do not enlarge on
how its goals can be achieved. According to Downie et al. (1990)
empowerment is the key. Health education is a way of empowering
people by providing them with information, and help in developing
their skills. This then allows them to feel that they have control
regarding their own health, resulting in a higher level of self esteem.
Nutbeam (1986) identifies self empowerment as being a process

which is designed to equip individuals with decision-making capabilities, enabling them to be autonomous.

In order for people to be empowered, health promotion must be concerned with broader issues such as the environment, preventive services and the formulation of policies. Individuals cannot be empowered without education, resources and processes within the community and environment, which will allow them to make the choice they want (Green and Raeburn, 1988; Kickbusch 1981; Saan 1986; Tannahill 1990; Tones 1983). Empowerment for the rehabilitation client should include:

- equal opportunities in the areas of employment, education and recreation
- adequate resources to allow them to return to their own environment
- equal access in the environment as people who are not disabled.

Preventative services could include those activities related to the causes of impairment, for example, screening for high blood pressure, family planning advice, stop smoking programmes, drink/driving laws and accident prevention.

Health education

Health education is often confused with health promotion. Does this matter? It could be said that there is no valid reason for distinguishing between health education and promotion. However, I would argue that nurses cannot adopt a philosophy of health promotion if they do not understand its principles, and its relationship to health education.

The role of health education is to ensure that people are knowledgeable and competent to allow them to be involved in the decision-making process. It helps individuals develop the skills that are needed to bring about change. Three stages of health education are described in the literature (Ewles and Simnett 1992; Tones 1981), primary, secondary and tertiary. The primary stage is concerned with the prevention of the onset of disease, secondary with the development of disease, and tertiary with rehabilitation. The tertiary stage is involved in enabling the individual to resume as full a life as possible, despite residual impairment; to abandon 'sick role' behaviour and accept 'healthy status'. Healthy status for the rehabilitation client could be interpreted as the achievement of their maximum potential, and a high level of wellbeing. Health education at this stage is concerned with providing clients with the skills and knowledge to enable them to resume former roles in life.

Maben and Macleod Clark (1995), following a conceptual analysis, summarise the concerns of health promotion and its relationship to health education as in Box 9.1.

Box 9.1
Health promotion

- is concerned with the prevention of disease
- is an attempt to improve the health status of an individual or community
- at its broadest level, is concerned with policies and legislation: the wider influences on health
- is dependent on health education which through information-giving, advice, support and skills training, attempts to raise awareness of the issue in question and fosters an ability to cope with illness or disease. Health education can be identified as being a necessary pre-requisite to health promotion
- is an approach to care through empowerment, equity, collaboration and participation, and may involve social and environmental change.

(Maben and Macleod Clark, 1995)

Health promotion and rehabilitation

According to Teague et al. (1990), the aim of rehabilitation is at the heart of all care provided to individuals with disabilities. This has resulted in a more advanced service, in the form of effective intervention strategies and better planning and coordination of services. However, these advances have not included comprehensive health promotion programmes. Teague et al. (1990) deliberate that this may be due to a lack of framework for applying the terms 'prevention' and 'promotion' to rehabilitation objectives and strategies.

Is the absence of a framework the only reason for this lack of emphasis on health promotion in rehabilitation, or does disability, with its devastating effects, cause barriers to health promotion? Stuifergen, Becker and Sands (1990) carried out a study of 135 disabled people to identify barriers which prevented them from improving and maintaining their own health. 47% of the sample listed either a neuro-cognitive or neuro-sensory impairment as their primary disability. Interestingly, when respondents were asked for their definitions of health, there was little mention of their disabilities. The majority emphasised a more functional or self-actualised definition of health, such as being independent or leading a normal life. Some respondents focused on what one needs to stay healthy, such as rest and exercise. A broad array of barriers were identified including their own motivation, their disability and lack of money. Stuifergen et al. (1990) concluded that health-promoting behaviour should receive as much emphasis for people with disabilities as other forms of life and work-skills training. Therefore, interventions aimed at decreasing barriers to health promotion would enhance an individual's quality of life, and could reduce the costs of health care for disabled people. The aim of health promotion is not to save money, but in the present economical climate it cannot be ignored.

However, it would be unethical if the main aim of incorporating health promotion programmes for disabled people was for financial gain.

Marge (1988) describes the major objectives underlying health maintenance strategies for people with disabilities as being to teach them to become personally responsible for their own health, and to co-manage their own rehabilitation programme. This view is supported by Price (1986), who in his model of rehabilitation identified the education programme as being designed to give clients increasing control over their own progress and health. Health promotion programmes for individuals with disabilities should be an essential part of the rehabilitation process, beginning in the primary treatment phase and continuing throughout life (Marge, 1988). In order for this to happen, rehabilitation professionals need to focus on health rather than disability.

Health can be viewed as a positive state of wellbeing, physically, socially and mentally and not merely as the absence of illness or disease (Downie et al., 1990; Clarke and Lowe, 1989; Tones, 1990). This definition has similarities with the traditional medical model, which views health as the absence of disease or infirmity. Both of these definitions leave little room for the disabled person to be considered healthy. It could be said that the medical model is not conducive to the aims of rehabilitation, yet it is this view that rehabilitation settings are generally adopting. Health promotion and rehabilitation are both concerned with health and wellness (Duffy, 1988; Marge, 1988). Beckman-Murray and Proctor Zentner (1989) identify that health-wellbeing and disease-illness, can be thought of as complex, dynamic processes on a continuum that includes physical, psychological, spiritual and social components. Wellness and hence health can exist independently of disability and disease, for example, a disabled person may be considered healthy within the limitations imposed on them by their disability.

According to the literature (Brandon, 1985; Marge, 1988; Teague et al., 1990), health promotion programmes for disabled people should include the following areas: principles of self-responsibility including self control, nutritional awareness, physical fitness, stress management, injury prevention, avoiding toxic substances and monitoring health status. There do not appear to be any differences between these programmes and health promotion programmes for people who are not disabled. However, if disabled people are to have the opportunity to resume former roles, these programmes are essential.

Nurse's role in health promotion

Faulkener (1984) suggests that health education should be an integral part of the nurse's role, being interpreted in terms of the physical, social and psychological welfare of the client. Nurses require the skills to assess a client's health problems and to plan, implement, and evaluate any intervention. Communication is identified as the main skill, being used as a basis for assessment and teaching. Do nurses have the skills? Latter et al. (1992) used a postal questionnaire survey of 142 senior nurses to gain their perceptions of health education activities on acute general wards. The survey results suggest that although clients may receive information from nurses, they are not necessarily being encouraged to participate in their care. Latter et al. (1992) suggests that a different philosophy is required if clients are to participate.

This view is supported by Lindsey and Hartrick (1996) who identify the tension between health promotion and the nursing process, which is based on a biomedical approach. They conclude that in order for nurses to adopt a health promotion approach, they need to examine their philosophy of care and their use of the nursing process, so that they make the shift from the natural science paradigm from which the nursing process emerged to the human science paradigm which focuses on the person's experiences of health.

A study by Eardley, Davis and Wakefield (1975) of 60 colostomy clients illustrated the difficulties involved when the responsibility for educating clients towards better health is not recognised. The study highlighted the need for one-to-one education, for improved communication within the team, and for training the doctors and nurses in the skills required for educating clients. The study concluded that health education for clients with chronic illness or disability should be regarded as a vital part of treatment and as such, is an important nursing role. Although an old study, based on my own experience I would suggest that the problems have not changed.

Group work, individual instruction and giving of written and visual information are strategies which nurses can use in the delivery of health education (Coutts and Hardy, 1985; Ewles and Simnett, 1992). The nurse as a role model can be identified as another strategy. Clarke (1991) argues that nurses' credibility is not necessarily related to their own health-related activities. Slater (1990) suggests that nurses should aim to be effective role models, by concentrating on areas such as personal effectiveness, confidence in self, and communication. Coutts and Hardy (1985) advocate that nurses can help solve health related problems by informing, advising and assisting in the areas listed in Box 9.2

Box 9.2
Areas in which nurses can inform, advise and assist

- the acquisition of skills
- the clarification of feelings, beliefs and values
- the client's and family's adaptation of lifestyle
- the promotion of change in the organisations which influence health status
- the provision of a model of values and behaviours related to health

(Coutts and Hardy, 1985)

The role of the nurse in rehabilitation can be identified as being to help clients adapt to the changes associated with their impairment and disability, and to teach them more efficient ways of coping with every-day demands. Diehl (1989) identifies the goals of rehabilitation nursing as being to prevent further impairment, to monitor existing ability, and to restore as much function as possible. I would suggest that these goals come within the remit of health promotion, with health education providing the teaching component. Teaching is recognised in the literature as being an important element of the rehabilitation nurse's role, instrumental in helping client and family adapt to changes (Baker, 1990; DeVito, 1988; Power, 1989; Wade, Lemermann and Mastroanni, 1983; White and Holloway, 1990).

Diehl (1989) emphasises the importance of collaborative goal setting with clients and their families, which is also a characteristic of the interdisciplinary team. Kowalsky (1985) emphasises the rehabilitation nurse's role in the health maintenance of clients, identifying dental care, nutrition, physical activity, safety and counseling as being essential to any programme. Assessment, as well as including physical independence in meeting personal health needs, should include the client's readiness and ability to learn. Their social situation should be taken into account, as well as feelings and knowledge regarding their condition, interests and aspirations (Kowalsky 1985; Syred 1981; Wilhide Tanner, 1991).

Rehabilitation nurse's role in health promotion

From the literature, the rehabilitation nurse's role in health promotion can be summarised as follows:

- Helping clients and their families adapt.

Rehabilitation clients are undergoing constant change due to their disabilities, and may need support in the form of counseling and coping strategies.

- Assessment to include client's knowledge base, their feelings, interests and aspirations.

Assessment must include these aspects, if the nurse is to formulate effective health promotion programmes with the client.

- Setting client-centred goals with the client, family and the interdisciplinary team.

If clients are to be empowered, goals regarding their rehabilitation need to be set collaboratively

- Teaching clients and families.

Clients will need to be taught different skills to enable them to be as independent as possible. Families may require instruction in how to help their relative.

■ Helping clients in health maintenance activities.

In particular, activities such as: dental hygiene which clients may not be able to deal with effectively; nutrition and physical fitness because clients may not be as active, and may need to adapt their diet and physical exercise; safety, where clients need to be made aware of their limitations and taught ways of coping if they fall, for example.

The views in the literature are substantiated by the results from my own small qualitative study (Davis, 1995) which explored the nurse's understanding of health education and health promotion and their role within it, and their perception of illness and wellness related to disability. This study was conducted at two neuro-rehabilitation centres in England using 18 questionnaires, 3 group interviews and content analysis of 39 client care plans. Although the nurses had difficulty distinguishing between health promotion and health education, differences did emerge which were supported by the literature. The nurses identified health promotion as covering all aspects of their role. Constraints to this role included using a problem-oriented approach, and lack of knowledge. The content analysis of the care plans supported a lack of a health promotion ethos in the language used.

The main premise of the study was that rehabilitation nurses were attempting to encourage, teach and involve clients in their care, in

Figure 9.1
Health promotion model for rehabilitation nursing

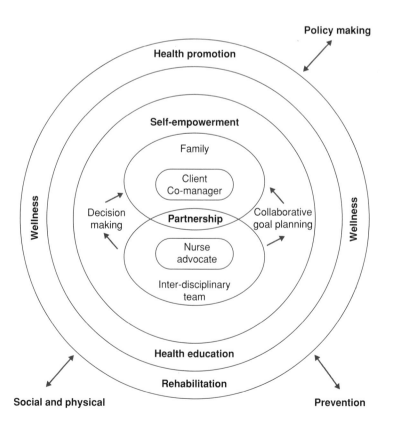

an ethos of disability, rather than wellness. The results support this. Generally, wellness was equated with physical independence. As a result of the study, I was able to develop the following health promotion model (see also Fig. 9.1) which is based on the principles of self-empowerment. Although the study was directed at nurses working in neuro-rehabilitation, I would suggest that this model could be used as a framework for rehabilitation nurses and other professionals in any area of health care, to enable them to focus on health and wellness rather than illness and disability.

Health promotion

Ultimately, health promotion and rehabilitation are concerned with promoting wellness. A disabled person can be considered healthy within the limitations imposed on them by their disability. To enable disabled individuals to have a sense of wellbeing and be considered healthy, the issues in Box 9.3 need to be addressed.

Box 9.3
Issues to address for wellbeing and health

> **Social and physical environment**
> Access to leisure facilities
> The same access in the environment as non-disabled people
> Adequate support services and resources, to enable individuals to return to their own environment
> Support groups in the community, for clients and families
> Support for employers to enable disabled individuals to return to work
> **Prevention**
> Active enforcement of seat belt and drink/driving laws
> Stronger penalties for drink driving
> Screening for high blood pressure
> Family planning advice
> Education on diet, alcohol, drugs, smoking and accident prevention
> **Policy Making**
> Equal opportunities policies for disabled people
> Policies related to alcohol and tobacco advertising
> Policies related to new buildings

Nurses have a role in promoting the issues in Box 9.3, in being involved in lobbying for changes in policies and the environment, actively complaining about inadequate facilities for disabled people, being involved in support groups in the community and encouraging and enabling disabled individuals and their families to be involved. Nurses should also have an understanding of relevant legislation affecting disabled people such as the Disability Discrimination Act (1995).

Health Education   The aim of health education, within health promotion, is to empower individuals by providing them with information and decision-making skills. In rehabilitation, health education activities include those listed in Box 9.4.

Box 9.3
Health education
activities

> **Promotion of independence**
> Self-care activities, for example, washing, dressing, feeding, communication
> Collaborative goal planning with the client, family and the rest of the team
> Instructing the client and their relatives
>
> **Adaptation to lifestyle**
> Counselling including sexual counselling
> Psychological support
> Teaching new skills
> Managing stress
>
> **Health maintenance**
> Nutrition, dental hygiene, and physical exercise
> Avoidance of toxic substances, for example, smoking, drugs and alcohol
> Management of epilepsy
> Monitoring blood pressure and blood glucose

A variety of strategies can be used to convey information including one-to-one interaction, visual information, group sessions, and individual and group health programmes.

Client   Within this health promotion model, clients are identified as being co-managers of their rehabilitation programmes, with a certain amount of control over their own health. The amount of control may vary depending on other factors, for example, the environment, other people and the client's degree of disability. Even clients with severe disability are able to have some control of their life. The philosophy of self-empowerment for these clients should remain the same.

The family is recognised as being an important part of the client's life. It must be the client's decision if this is different. Clients have choices concerning their life and the changes they are experiencing. In order for them to be able to make informed decisions, they require support from the nurses and the rest of the interdisciplinary team. Their relationship with the nurses is one of partnership. Assertiveness training, and decision-making skills should be available to the client to enable them to achieve self-empowerment.

Nurse   The nurse's role is one of advocacy, and informing and supporting clients to enable them to make decisions. As suggested by Teague et al (1990), the rehabilitation nurse can be identified as a collaborator, educator and provider of health promotion programmes. The nurses also have a responsibility in communicating effectively with the rest of the team, and in continually improving their knowledge base. In order to assume these roles, nurses need to be skilled in assessment, communication, counselling, teaching, negotiation and facilitation. The nurses' concern includes involvement in the activities mentioned under health education and health promotion. Nurses need to ensure that their approach to planning care is conducive to the concepts of health promotion. For example, the problem-solving approach of the nursing process may not enhance interdisciplinary goal setting and the involvement of clients in decision-making (this is discussed in more detail in chapter 6).

Conclusion

The common factor between health promotion and rehabilitation relates to wellness. Rehabilitation should be concerned with health rather than disability and the main aim of health promotion is to promote health. It would then appear feasible that rehabilitation programmes adopt more of a health promotion approach. The definitions of health promotion and health education discussed, appear to agree that health promotion is concerned with broader, societal issues, such as the formulation of policies and the environment. The aim of health promotion programmes is to empower people so that they are able to sustain or increase their level of wellbeing. Health education is an information-giving activity which empowers people by helping them develop decision-making skills.

If clients are to become personally responsible for their own health and to co-manage their rehabilitation programme, then health promotion needs to be at the heart of rehabilitation. Nurses are in the ideal position to include health promotion in their practice. One could argue that the rehabilitation nurse's role is primarily one of health promotion. Aspects of the role identified in the literature would support this view, as would the results from my own study. The suggested health promotion model could be used as a framework on which to base practice and improve client care. It could assist in improving clients' care by enabling them to have self empowerment, and subsequently self-esteem, and to enable rehabilitation professionals to focus on wellness, rather than disability.

Questions for discussion

- What is the focus of rehabilitation in your area?

- How can you promote a health promotion focus?

- What would be the advantages or disadvantages to your clients of using a framework such as the one described?

References

Baker, J. E. (1990) Family adaption when one member has a head injury. *Journal of Neuroscience Nursing*, 22, 232–237.

Beckman Murray, R. & Procter Zentner, J. (1989) *Nursing Concepts for Health Promotion*. London: Prentice-Hall.

Brandon, J. E. (1985) Health promotion and wellness in rehabilitation services. *Journal of Rehabilitation*, **51**, 54–58.

Clarke, A. C. (1991) Nurses as role models and health educators. *Journal of Advanced Nursing*, **16**, 1178–1184.

Clarke, R. & Lowe, F. (1989) Positive health – some lay perspectives. *Health Promotion*, **3**, 401–406.

Coutts, L. C. & Hardy, L. K. (1985) *The Nurse as Health Educator*. London: Churchill Livingstone.

Davis, S. M. (1995) An investigation into nurses' understanding of health education and health promotion within a neuro-rehabilitation setting. *Journal of Advanced Nursing*, **21**, 951–959.

DeVito, A. J. (1988) Documenting client education in rehabilitation: an interdisciplinary approach. *Rehabilitation Nursing*, **13**, 26–28.

Diehl, L. N. (1989) Client and family learning in the rehabilitation setting. *Nursing Clinics of North America*, **24**, 257–264.

Downie, R. S., Fyfe, C. & Tannahill, A. (1990) *Health Promotion: Models and Values*. Oxford: Oxford University Press.

Duffy, M. E. (1988) Health promotion in the family: current findings and directives for nursing research. *Journal of Advanced Nursing*, **13**, 109–117.

Eardley, A. Davis, J. & Wakefield, J. (1975) Health education by chance – the unmet needs of patients in hospital and after. *International Journal of Health Education*, **18**, 19–25.

Ewles, L. and Simnett, I. (1992) *Promoting Health: A Practical Guide*, 2nd edn. London: Scutari Press.

Faulkener, A. (1984) Health education in nursing. *Nursing Times*, **80**, 45–46.

Green, L. W. & Raeburn, J. M. (1988) *Health Promotion*, **3**, 151–159.

Henderson, V. & Nite, G. (1978) *Principles and Practice of Nursing*. New York: Macmillan Publishing Co.

Kickbusch, I. (1981) Involvement in health – a social concept of health education. *International Journal of Health Education and Supplement*, **24**, 1–15.

Kowalsky, E. L. (1985) The nurse's role in health maintenance of the physically disabled client. *Rehabilitation Nursing*, **10**, 9–12.

Latter, S., Macleod Clark, J., Wilson Barnett, J. & Maben, J. (1992) Health education in nursing: perceptions of practice in acute settings. *Journal of Advanced Nursing*, **17**, 164–172.

Lindsey, E. & Hartrick, G. (1996) Health-promoting nursing practice: the demise of the nursing process? *Journal of Advanced Nursing*, **23**, 106–112.

Maben, J. & Macleod Clark, J. (1995) Health promotion: a concept analysis. *Journal of Advanced Nursing*, **22**, 1158–1165.

Marge, M. (1988) Health promotion for persons with disabilities: moving beyond rehabilitation. *American Journal of Health Promotion*, **2**, 29–35.

Melvin, J. L. (1989) Status report of inter-disciplinary medical rehabilitation. *Archives of Physical Medicine and Rehabilitation*, **70**, 273–276.

Nutbeam, D. (1986) Health promotion glossary. *Health Promotion*, **1**, 113–127.

Pender, N. J. (1987) *Health Promotion in Nursing Practice*, 2nd edn. Norwalk: CT Appleton and Lange.

Power, P. W. (1989) Working with families: an intervention model for rehabilitation nurses. *Rehabilitation Nursing*, **14**, 73–76.

Price, B. (1986) Giving the patient control. *Nursing Times*, **82**, 28–30.

Saan, H. (1986) Health promotion and health education: living with a dominant concept. *Health Promotion*, **1**, 253–255.

Slatter, J. (1990) Effecting personal effectiveness: assertiveness training for nurses. *Journal of Advanced Nursing*, **15**, 337–356.

Stuifergen, A. K., Becker, H. & Sands, D. (1990) Barriers to health promotion for individuals with disabilities. *Community Health*, **13**, 11–22.

Syred, M. E. J. (1981) The abdication of the role of health education by hospital nurses. *Journal of Advanced Nursing*, **6**, 27–33.

Tannahill, A. (1985) What is health promotion?

Health Education Journal **44**, 167–168.

Tannahill, A. (1990) Health education and health promotion: planning for the 1990s. *Health Education Journal*, **49**, 194–198.

Teague, M. L., Cipriano, R. E. & McGhee, V. L. (1990) Health promotion as a rehabilitation service for people with disabilities. *Journal of Rehabilitation*, **56**, 52–56.

Tones, B. K. (1981) Prevention or subversion? *Royal Society of Health Journal*, **101**, 114–117.

Tones, B. K. (1983) Education and health promotion: new direction. *Journal of the Institute of Health Education*, **21**, 121–131.

Wade, N. P., Lemerman, R. D. & Mastroianni, E. J. (1983) Rehabilitative care and education. Practical guidelines for preparing patients to function at home. *Rehabilitation Nursing*, **8**, 32–35.

Wade, D. T. (1996) *Rivermead Report Number Eight*. Oxford: Parchment (Oxford) Ltd.

White, M. J. & Holloway, M. (1990) Patient concerns after discharge from rehabilitation. *Rehabilitation Nursing*, **15**, 316–318.

Wilhide Tanner, E. K. (1991) Assessment of a health-promotive lifestyle. *Nursing Clinics of North America*, **26**, 845–854.

World Health Organisation (1980) *International Classification of Impairments, Disabilities and Handicaps (ICIDH)*. Geneva: WHO.

World Health Organisation (1986) Ottawa Charter for Health Promotion. *Journal of Health Promotion*, **1**, 1–14.

Location of care

Stephen O'Connor, Gill Weaver

Key issues

- Stroke nursing in general units
- Potential problems of stroke wards
- An atmosphere conducive to care
- Community links

Introduction

The term 'location of care' is taken to mean the broad social and environmental surroundings within which care is delivered. The arguments regarding the location in which care is delivered are the subject matter of this chapter. The central theme is that the correct location and environment are important, if not a prerequisite, to the ability of nurses to deliver the nursing care that they consider appropriate. The three sections that make up this chapter are, first, the perceived problems of delivering nursing care to stroke patients in an acute ward, secondly, the potential difficulties of dedicated stroke units and thirdly, the perceived atmosphere of a ward that nurses and their clients would regard as appropriate. The conclusion will draw out the principles, for rehabilitation in general, of the importance of dedicated areas and the care which can be delivered. These sections illuminate the factors of a distinctive ward area dedicated to rehabilitation care, and a particular atmosphere that is seen as a requisite to the rehabilitation of clients, which is created by the nurses. Discussion centres around the benefits of dedicated units in the rehabilitation of stroke patients. This area of rehabilitation has been chosen as the literature is extensive on the evaluation of stroke units as opposed to any other form of rehabilitation centre. The chapter will also be illustrated by a number of sketches of rehabilitation units, to demonstrate the diversity of locations that cover rehabilitative care. (see Boxes 10.1–10.3).

Box 10.1
A rehabilitation location for amputees

The XXXXXXXX rehabilitation unit is a specialised inpatient service and follow-up outreach service designed for the rehabilitation of amputees following a brief 5-day surgical episode undertaken in two general vascular wards of the local general hospital.

The purpose-built unit, 5 miles from the general hospital in a country setting, was sited on the ground floor with an integral therapy department for the ongoing delivery of both physiotherapy and occupational therapy, which provided input of up to 3 days a week for each client. In 1996, the outreach service was introduced, which allowed the clients to be cared for in the community at an earlier stage of their rehabilitation.

The unit allows for the delivery of appropriate care from specialist nurses, in terms of quicker, more focused specialist nursing care and a streamlined service in relation to the fitting and delivery of the clients' prostheses. The unit has led to less anxiety on the part of clients about returning home, given the full support of the team. The improved prosthesis service has led to an improved standard of mobility and normal functioning for the amputees.

The impact on nursing staff has been considerable, not only in terms of the need for full team commitment to individualised rehabilitation goals over the 24-hour period, but also the need for staff to take a step back from the traditional 'doing' role to the more appropriate 'enabling'. This change of emphasis has only been made possible by an investment in staff training and education.

Stroke nursing in general units

Research carried out into the nursing care of stroke clients admitted to general medical wards demonstrates a consistent picture of poor care delivered by' staff who are poorly motivated, and at best, ambivalent towards stroke clients. Stockwell (1972), in a study of nurses' attitudes towards various types of clients on general medical wards found that stroke clients were categorised in the 'unpopular patient' group.

Characteristics such as protracted duration of stay, uncooperativeness, difficulties with nurse–client communication and the perception that stroke clients were unlikely to progress, were perceived as characteristic. Hamrin (1982), in a study of four general medical wards and Gibbon (1991), in a similarly structured study, both demonstrated that nurses, regardless of their status and training, were likewise, at best, ambivalent towards stroke clients. In an observational study of the care delivered to stroke clients on a medical ward, Patrick (1972), in an article entitled 'Forgotten Patients on the Medical Ward', identified that few nurses provided conditions in which clients could attempt to manage their own activities of living unaided. Furthermore, clients were frequently left in chairs for prolonged periods, bowel and bladder regimes were not seen as important and exercise was seldom included in stroke client care.

The majority of research has been undertaken in acute areas in the sphere of community care, and a similar picture is to be seen here. Kratz (1978) describes a picture of nurses who ascribe value to their care only when they can see the direct value of that care in terms of demonstrable outcomes. Therefore, the value perceived in the care of stroke clients is that attributed to the acute stage of the disease when the client is seriously ill, or later, in the disease process when the client's improvements can be observed. This implies that the care required by stroke clients when their condition is improving slowly or has stabilized is not valued. Gibbon (1993), in a study of community nurses, identified a similar picture in which district nurses did not perceive themselves as having a role in stroke rehabilitation; their interventions were concerned with the effects of chronicity. Hence, when a stroke client's condition deteriorated to the extent that they or their carer could no longer manage their activity of living needs, then the nurse (usually an auxiliary nurse) would become involved in a supportive manner.

Overall, these articles paint a gloomy picture of nurses who do not appreciate the needs of stroke clients, do not appreciate their role in caring for stroke clients and have little understanding of the meaning or the concept of rehabilitation. The explanation for the situation is consistently seen as being either lack of time to spare for stroke clients (Gibbon, 1993; Hamrin, 1982; Patrick, 1972) or lack of expertise or awareness (Gibbon, 1994; Patrick, 1972). However, as both Hamrin (1982) and Gibbon (1991) demonstrate, the provision of educational packages for nurses does not produce a significant improvement in client care over those nurses that do not receive such education.

The evaluation of stroke units

The beneficence of rehabilitation in stroke care has been well described in the literature (Aitken, Rogers and French, 1993; Feigenson, 1981; Feldman, Lee and Unterecker, 1962; Hamrin, 1982; Lehmann, Delateur and Fowler, 1975; Smith et al., 1981). The claim made by the proponents of stroke units is that the care of the stroke client is significantly better in demonstrable terms than that delivered in other care areas (Drummond, Lincoln and Juby, 1996; Edmans and Towle, 1990; Garraway et al., 1980a, 1980b; Indredavik et al., 1991; Juby, Lincoln & Berman, 1996; Kalra, 1994; Kalra, Dale and Crome, 1993; Stevens, Ambler and Warren, 1984; Strand et al., 1985, 1986; Von Arbin et al., 1979, 1980). The belief that care is better given in a stroke unit was initially not proven, because the evaluations did not fulfil the criteria for medical research, i.e. random prospective controlled trial (Garraway, 1985). The positive evaluations that were put forward were disregarded as not demonstrating the therapeutic value of stroke units in acceptable terms (Langton-Hewer, & Holbrook, 1983; Orgogozo, Castel and Dartigues, 1982; Von Arbin et al., 1980). The first major trial was that of Garraway et al., (1980a and 1980b), which although initially demonstrating a benefit of a stroke unit over a general medical unit, on follow-up, found that the comparative improvement was not sustained over time.

More trials carried out in the UK and Sweden have demonstrated both that the outcomes are initially demonstrable and that these benefits last over time (Drummond et al., 1996; Edmans and Towle, 1990; Indredavik et al., 1991; Juby et al., 1996; Kalra, 1994; Kalra et al. 1993; Stevens et al. 1984; Strand et al. 1985, 1986).

In addition to these trials, two important meta-analyses have been carried out regarding stroke rehabilitation. The first was undertaken by Ottenbacher and Jannell (1993) and addressed the effect of stroke rehabilitation programmes in general. Out of 124 research reports addressed, 36 trials met the criteria for inclusion as being randomised, controlled trials. The analysis therefore covered 3717 clients and demonstrated that the average client allocated to a stroke programme performed better than 65% of those clients in comparable groups. The second mata-analysis was undertaken by Langhorne et al. (1993) and investigated the specific effect of designated stroke units on client outcome. Langhorne et al. identified 10 trials, eight of which they considered to have undertaken strict randomisation procedures. The analysis therefore covered 1586 clients and demonstrated that the:

> 'Management of stroke patients in a stroke unit is associated with a sustained reduction in mortality.'
>
> (Langhorne et al., 1993)

In relation to morbidity, Langhorne states that although all the studies demonstrate improvements in functional activity and none show poorer outcomes, a more detailed analysis was impossible due to the various outcome measures used in the studies.

Langhorne also addresses the potential problem of publication bias on the reliability of meta-analysis. The possibility that trials that found no change, or even poorer outcomes, were not published has to be taken into account. Langhorne takes the stance that the number of negative or neutral trials that would be required to significantly alter the overall findings of the meta-analysis would need to involve 1600 clients. Langhorne identified several trials in progress at the time of their analysis and anticipated that even if all these trials reported neutral results, the overall findings would still not be affected. In fact two of these trials, Kalra et al. (1993) in the Kent study and Juby et al. (1996) and Drummond et al. (1996) in the Nottingham study, support the findings of the Langhorne meta-analysis.

Potential problems of stroke wards

The very success of stroke units can also be seen as a cause of some concern, in that the expectations of both client and carers are raised by the existence of a specialist unit. A transfer to a stroke unit will act to raise the expectations of the carers of the clients with regard to the potential of the client, once on the stroke unit. In many instances, a general awareness amongst the staff on feeder wards that the client's potential is more likely to be achieved on the local stroke ward than anywhere else adds to this level of expectation. It must be said, however, that stroke units are frequently seen as providing a convenient outlet for acute wards to move on those clients that they are no longer able to care for as positively as might be wished. The nurses on the acute wards are handicapped by the fact that they rarely see the final outcome of a successful rehabilitation process, as the clients are nearly always moved on as soon as possible to make way for more acute clients. This can be considered as a major disincentive to the nurses on the acute wards.

An atmosphere conducive to care

The atmosphere on a stroke ward, and the effects that the correct atmosphere has on the staff's ability to deliver the type of care that they feel appropriate, are important. The nurses' 24-hour presence, and the time available during the longer client stays, should be seen as precursors through which the right atmosphere can be created.

The atmosphere, while being relaxed and informal, must at the same time be structured and safe. The key concepts that define the required ward are friendly, relaxed, homely and deliberately low-stress. These concepts would appear to paint a picture of a rather liberal regime, however this cannot be the case. The atmosphere is required to be like this so that the process of rehabilitation can be facilitated, as a strict regime would be counter-productive, however, the regime cannot be too liberal either. The ward regime should have strict boundaries that ensure that the environment on the ward, while relaxed and even 'laid back' remains controlled, structured and safe.

The balance between these two potentially disparate interpretations is important and would seem to indicate that while other wards are inhibited by their acute nature, which necessitates a close attachment to routine, stroke wards use routine to maintain a discipline in the care process, but are able to be much more flexible than acute wards can be. Boundaries are set by various mechanisms. Professional standards have to be maintained regardless of the degree of relaxation and the environment has to be safe and secure, in that protocols of care are adhered to, so as to uphold safety during risk-taking procedures.

The nurses' task is to create the right atmosphere on the ward. There are two mechanisms at work that should help towards the creation of the ward environment. First, the ward environment is created by the intentional activity of the nurses to promote such an atmosphere and is therefore manufactured. The creation of the right ward environment by the nurses is very important, it should be seen as a priority. Orem describes providing a developmental environment as one of the five key actions within the Methods of Assisting

(Orem, 1991). In essence, this implies that the nurses are responsible for the provision of an environment conducive to the client's recover.

Box 10.2
British Home and Hospital, London

British Home and Hospital, London, provides long-term, short-term and respite care for people with neurological and other physical disabilities, and chronic illness.

Care is aimed at preserving function and therefore independence. Preventing further deterioration in health is very important because of the long-term nature of disability, but when chronic illness progresses, the residents are taught adaptation and compensation. The person's abilities and life experiences are valued by the staff and help to provide the basis of a creative working relationship.

Residents have access to nursing and medical services, physiotherapy, social and recreational activities, dental, optical and chiropody services and counselling.

Staff work with residents to encourage and promote independence while providing skilled, intensive nursing care to people with greater needs. The emphasis of the nursing care is on activities of daily living. Many residents have particular needs in the prevention of the undesirable effects of immobility, incontinence and dysphagia. The psychosocial aspects of nursing care are mainly to help with cognitive deficits and to assist development of attitudes necessary to lead a constructive and fulfilled life within the limitations caused by illness.

The second factor is that the clients are on the same ward for longer and therefore the nurses have more time with them. Clients spend more time on stroke wards than they do on acute wards. However, the overall length of stay for stroke clients is less on the dedicated stroke wards than on any other ward where stoke clients receive their rehabilitation (Strand et al., 1985). The length of stay on the ward is sufficient to allow the staff to get to know the clients and their relatives better than on acute wards, where the majority of stroke clients still spend most of their time while in hospital. The length of stay and the acceptance of a slower, more relaxed pace must be seen as central to the production of the correct atmosphere for the rehabilitation process. The creation of the friendly, supportive environment may therefore be seen as a by-product of the fact that the nurses are able to get to know the clients better because they are on the ward longer than is the case on acute wards.

Overall, the creation of the ward atmosphere must therefore be seen as an important aspect of the nurse's role, and a prerequisite for the delivery of the care that the nurses must deliver. The atmosphere of the ward should be seen by nurses as their responsibility, nurses need to create a relaxed and informal atmosphere, at the same time retaining adequate control over the ward so as to maintain a safe and professionally-organised ward environment.

Community links

An understanding of the locality which a stroke unit serves, along with a close liaison with the local community staff and a commitment to post-discharge involvement in the clients' ongoing care are all important to rehabilitation care. A knowledge is required not only of the local population but also the local services available and the pathways that clients can negotiate to get the best care. A knowledge of the local community staff is similarly required to both smooth the discharge of a client back to the community and to ensure that the community staff are aware of the needs of the client.

Box 10.3
Rivermead Rehabilitation Centre

Rivermead Rehabilitation Centre in Oxford is a neurological centre admitting clients from Oxfordshire, neighbouring counties and further afield. The main criteria for admission to Rivermead is that clients have to be medically stable and be able to participate to a degree in the rehabilitation process.

The majority of clients at Rivermead are aged between 20 and 70 years and have suffered either a stroke or head injury. Clients present with a range of disabilities including physical, cognitive and behavioural. Rivermead has 30 beds plus a large number of outpatient places. The team consists of doctors, qualified and unqualified nurses, physiotherapists, occupational therapists, social workers, clinical psychologists, speech and language therapists and a psychiatrist.

Rivermead uses an interdisciplinary approach, with the focus being on goal planning. All clients complete a life goals questionnaire to ensure a focus on the level of handicap. This is then used to identify the aims of their individualised rehabilitation programme. Clients then have an individualised programme according to their needs, which if appropriate, will include access to the leisure project. Regular reviews are held for each client to review life goals, progress and aims.

The length of stay for clients at Rivermead varies, being on average between 3 and 6 months for people following stroke, and up to a year for people with head injury. However, discharge is often delayed due to lack of community resources.

The need for post-hospital involvement and the accompanying local liaison is a distinctive feature of the full process of care. However, the ability to fulfil that expectation can be compromised by a lack of facilities and finance as few budgets run to such ends. The commonest form of post-discharge follow-up care is the stroke club. These are opportunities for discharged clients to return to the ward or unit to meet other stroke clients and carers, discuss any problems they may have and perhaps meet and encourage new stroke victims setting out on their rehabilitation path. The voluntary nature of the clubs is a common feature but one that should be seen as correct, as the clients have been discharged and are therefore able to choose whether to attend. However, it is important that as many as possible do attend, so as to create a positive environment for new clients, as well as old. The need for respite on a frequent basis for the carer cannot be minimised. The need on the part of those expert in stroke care to be involved in preventative care is also an important aspect of the links with the community.

Conclusion

The existence of stroke units, as centres where nurses and other professionals can work in a situation which can allow for a slower pace, is central to the rehabilitation of stroke clients. The existence of stroke units facilitates the delivery of the correct care. The concentration of clients allows for the development of the nursing practices that could not be fully applied in areas where other commitments take priority. An ability to concentrate on the needs of stroke clients also allows for the continuity of care to stretch beyond the hospital environment, so as to improve the client's long-term care in the community. The atmosphere of the ward should be seen by nurses as their responsibility; they should create a relaxed and informal atmosphere but also retain adequate control over the ward, so as to maintain a safe and professionally-organised ward environment.

This chapter has dealt exclusively with the case of stroke units. This is because it is in this area that most research has been undertaken. With regard to other rehabilitation areas, the inclusion of the brief descriptions of rehabilitation units that care for other classes of clients (Boxes 10.1–10.3) goes some way to making the point that the nature of rehabilitation itself requires a location that will allow the specific form of care that nurses and other professionals wish to deliver, regardless of the client group. For the same reason that ITUs and CCUs separated from general surgical and medical wards, and care of the elderly wards separated from acute areas, so rehabilitation units developed in all clinical areas. The nature of rehabilitation nursing care requires a distinctive environment and atmosphere that can only be created by the nurses in a dedicated unit.

References

Aitken, P.D., Rogers, H. & French, J.M. (1993) General medical or geriatric unit care for acute stroke? *Age and Ageing*, **22** (suppl 2), 4–5.

Drummond, A., Lincoln, N.B. & Juby, L.C. (1996) Effects of a stroke unit on knowledge of stroke and experiences in hospital. *Health Trends*, **28**, 26–30.

Edmans, J.A. & Towle, D. (1990) Comparison of stroke unit and non-stroke unit inpatients on independence in ADL. *British Journal of Occupational Therapy*, **53**, 415–418.

Feigenson, J. (1981) Stroke rehabilitation. *Stroke*, **12**, 373–375.

Feldman, D.J., Lee, P.R. & Unterecker, J. (1962) A comparison of functionally orientated medical care and formal rehabilitation in the management of patients with hemiplegia due to cerebrovascular accident. *Journal of Chronic Disability*, **15**, 297–310.

Garraway, W. (1985) Stroke rehabilitation units: concepts, evaluation and unresolved issues. *Stroke*, **16**, 178–181.

Garraway, M., Akhtar, A., Prescott, R. & Hockey, L. (1980a) Management of acute stroke in the elderly: preliminary results of a controlled trial. *British Medical Journal*, **280**, 1040–1043.

Garraway, M., Akhtar, A., Hockey, L. & Prescott, R. (1980b) Management of acute stroke in the elderly: follow-up of a controlled trial. *British Medical Journal*, **281**, 827–829.

Gibbon, G. (1991) An assessment of nurses' attitudes towards stroke patients in general medical wards. *Journal of Advanced Nursing*, **16**, 1336–1342.

Gibbon, G. (1994) Stroke nursing care and management in the community: a survey of district nurses' perceived contribution in one health district in England. *Journal of Advanced Nursing*, **29**, 469–476.

Hamrin, E. (1982) One year after stroke: a follow-up of an experimental study. *Scandinavian Journal of Rehabilitation Medicine*, **14**, 111–116.

Indredavik, B., Bakke, F., Solberg, R., Rokseth, R., Haaheim, L. & Holme, I. (1991) Benefit of a stroke unit: a randomized controlled trial. *Stroke*, **22**, 1026–1031.

Juby, L.C. Lincoln, N.B. & Berman, P. (1996) The effect of stroke unit rehabilitation on functional and psychological outcome: a randomised controlled trial. *Cerebrovascular Disease*, **6**, 106–110.

Kalra, I. (1994) The influence of stroke unit rehabilitation on functional recovery from stroke. *Stroke*, **24**(4), 821–825.

Kalra, L., Dale, P. & Crome, P. (1993) Improving stroke rehabilitation: a controlled study. *Stroke*, **24**, 1462–1467.

Kratz, C. (1978) *Care of the Long Term Sick in the Community*. Edinburgh: Churchill Livingstone.

Langhorne, P. Williams, B. Gilchrist, W. & Howie, K. (1993) Do stroke units save lives? *The Lancet*, **342**, 395–398.

Langton-Hewer, R. & Holbrook, M. (1983) The Bristol Stroke Unit. *Health Trends*, **83**, 15–18.

Lehmann, J., Delateur, B. & Fowler, R. (1975) Stroke: does rehabilitation affect outcome? *Archives of Physical and Medical Rehabilitation*, **56**, 375–382.

Orem, R. (1991) *Nursing: Concepts and Practice*, 4th edn. New York: McGraw Hill.

Orgogozo, J. Castel, J. & Dartigues, J. (1982) A stroke unit in Bordeaux. In *Advances in Stroke Therapy*, ed. Rose, F. New York: Raven Press.

Ottenbacher, K. & Jannell, S. (1993) The results of clinical trials in stroke rehabilitation research. *Archives in Neurology*, **50**, 37–44.

Patrick, G. (1972) Forgotten patients on the medical wards. *The Canadian Nurse*, **68**, 27–31.

Smith, D.S., Goldenberg, E., Ashburn A., et al. (1981) Remedial therapy after stroke: a randomised controlled trial. *British Medical Journal*, **282**, 517–520.

Stevens, R., Ambler, N. & Warren, M. (1984) A randomized controlled trial of a stroke rehabilitation ward. *Age & Ageing*, **13**, 65–75.

Stockwell, F. (1972) *The Unpopular Patient*. London: Royal College of Nursing.

Strand, T., Asplund, K., Erikson, S., Hagg, E., Lithner, F. & Wester, P. (1985) A non-intensive stroke unit reduces functional disability and the need for long term hospitalisation. *Stroke*, **16**, 29–34.

Strand, T., Asplund, K., Erikson, S., Hagg, E., Lithner, F. & Wester, P. (1986) Stroke unit care: who benefits a comparison with general medical. *Stroke*, **17**, 377–381.

Von Arbin, M., Britton, M., de Faire, U., et al. (1979) A stroke unit in a medical department:

organisation and the first 100 patients. *Acta Medica Scandiravica* **205**, 231–235.

Von Arbin, M., Britton, M., de Faire, U., Helmers, C., Miah, K. & Murray, V. (1980) A study of stroke patients treated in a non intensive stroke unit. *Acta Medica Scandinavica* **208**, 81–85.

Further reading

The following sources relate to the latest material regarding the evaluation of stroke units.

Stroke Unit Trialists' Collaboration (1997) How do stroke units improve patient outcomes? A collaborative systematic review of the randomized trials. *Stroke*, **28**, 2139–2144.

Stroke Unit Trialists' Collaboration (1997) Collaborative systematic review of the randomized trials of organised inpatient (stroke unit) care after stroke. *BMJ*, **314**, 1151–1159.

Langhorne, P. & Dennis, M. eds. (1998) *Stroke Units: an Evidence Based Approach.* London: BMJ.

11 The specialist nurse in rehabilitation

Andy Elliott

Key issues
- Specialism
- Specialist nursing
- Scope of professional practice
- Rehabilitation nurse specialist

Introduction

The aim of this chapter is to stimulate discussion and future debate with regards to the term 'rehabilitation nurse specialist'. It will explore the following:

- Definition of terms, roles and responsibilities of the nurse specialist
- Specialist nursing within an advanced nursing practice framework
- Preparation and requirements of a specialist nurse
- Scope of professional practice: opportunities and implications for rehabilitation nurse specialists
- Rehabilitation nurse specialists: 'generalist' or 'specialist'?

The view put forward is an entirely personal one based on the author's experience in the fields of orthopaedic, trauma, rehabilitation and elderly medical nursing.

Nursing specialisation is not a new phenomenon (Appel, 1996; Hamric and Spross, 1989; Hunt and Wainwright, 1994; Miller 1995; Storr, 1988). Nursing rehabilitation has been developed as a specialism in its own right (Buchanan, 1992; Habel, 1993). The history of rehabilitation nursing has been discussed in detail in Chapter 2.

Specialism

With all today's nursing jargon, which has taken on a global perspective (perhaps compounding confusion), terms such as 'Nurse practitioner', 'clinical nurse practitioner', 'specialist nurse', 'clinical nurse specialist' 'advanced nurse practitioner' only serve to muddy the water. This is paradoxical, as such a collection of ill-defined terms appears to highlight a juvenile profession. The promotion of specialism in nursing is seen to be a key feature in the process of nursing moving from an occupational group to a true profession (Hunt and Wainwright, 1994). The terms could also be as a result of individual's personal egotism, elitism and intra-professional rivalry, some people seeking to be more than 'just a nurse'.

Over the past 10 years, there has been a proliferation of nurse specialist posts, i.e. diabetes, palliative care, rheumatology, etc. According to O'Hanlon and Gibbon (1996), some people in post are '. . . self-styled specialists who have had little or no formal development'. For those who did receive formal development courses, the literature reports that courses varied from 6 weeks to 2 years. Butterworth (1994) suggests that titles implying clinical expertise are given to nurses who do not practice; they are neither 'clinical' nor very 'special'. This, he feels, does a great disservice to those who are actually clinical specialists.

From the literature, it is apparent that the definition of specialism originally emanates from the USA. Specialist nursing is defined by many sources. According to Hoeffer and Murphy (1984), the American Nurses Association's definition of specialist nursing is:

> '. . a narrow focus on a part of the whole field of nursing. It entails the application of a broad range of theories to selected phenomenon within the domain of nursing, in order to secure depth of understanding as a basis for advances in nursing.'
>
> (Hoeffer and Murphy 1984, p. 1)

According to the International Council of Nurses (ICN), specialisation:

> '. . . implies a level of knowledge and skill in a particular aspect of nursing which is greater than that acquired in the course of basic education.'
>
> (ICN 1992, p. 2)

The Royal College of Nursing have described the function of the nurse specialist as being:

> 'to provide direct patient care and to influence other nurses in doing so.'
>
> (RCN, 1988, p. 7)

Wallace and Gough (1995) have described the United Kingdom Central Council for Nursings' definition for a clinical nurse specialist as:

> '. . . a practitioner who exercises a higher level of judgement and discretion in clinical care in order to function as a specialist nursing practitioner.'
>
> (Wallace and Gough, 1995, p. 939)

The ICN's position on nurse specialism is:

> 'The nurse specialist is a nurse prepared beyond the level of a nurse generalist and authorised to practice as a specialist with advanced nursing expertise in the field of nursing. Speciality

practice includes clinical, teaching, administration, research and consultant roles. Post-basic nursing education for speciality practice is a formally recognised programme of study built upon the general education of the nurse and providing the content and experience to ensure competence in speciality practice. Preparation and authorisation are in accordance with scope of practice and within the education and regularity policies and practices for post-basic specialists in other professions.'

(ICN, 1992, p. 12)

Specialist nursing

Many UK and Australian authors (Lunt 1995, Al Leh 1996) have commented on the role of the clinical nurse specialist. These comments appear to echo the sentiments of US authors (Vitello-Ciccui, 1984; Girard, 1987). It is generally recognised that the roles of the nurse specialist include those listed in Box 11.1.

Box 11.1
Roles of the nurse specialist

- Practitioner/clinician
- Teacher
- Consultant
- Change agent
- Researcher
- Staff advocate
- Clinical leader
- Manager/administrator

The roles identified in Box 11.1 can be encompassed in the model shown in Figure 11.1 (Ryan 1996).

Specialisation within the post-registration educational practice (PREP) framework (UKCC, 1994) is outlined in the clinical practice level model (Table 11.1) devised by Elliott (1997).

Interestingly, Nash (1993) suggests that the job descriptions of specialist nursing posts have often been left to the specialists to define. One could argue that it is highly appropriate for such professionals to define their own specialist roles; they, after all, are the clinical specialist. The ICN (1992) has produced guidance and criteria for nursing specialities (see Table 11.1).

Figure 11.1
Model of roles for the nurse specialist

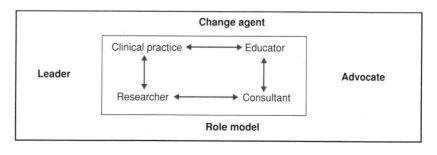

Table 11.1
Clinical practice level model (Elliott, 1997, with permission from Butterworth Heinemann)

Practice level	Educational level	Cognitive level	Skill level	Experiential level
Preceptored practice	Diploma (2) Degree (3)	Knowledge Comprehension	Novice: professional awareness	Exposure Participation
Professional practice	Degree (3) Masters (3)	Application	Competent: professional identity	Identification
Specialist practice	Diploma (2) Degree (M)	Analysis Synthesis	Proficient: professional maturity	Internalisation
Advanced practice	Masters (M) Doctorate (PhD)	Evaluation	Expert: professional mastery	Dissemination

Such an approach should be applauded, as nurse managers who encourage the approach in Table 11.1 demonstrate excellent leadership and vision. Sadly, this is not always the case. There are areas where such job descriptions are written, by 'managers' far removed from the situation, and with no significant speciality background. This is perhaps the 'hangover' effect of the days of paternalistic management, where nurses were 'compliant children' (Berne, 1984), and were told what to do, and when to do it. Hopefully this is slowly fading into the history of the profession.

The journey to true professional status is a rocky road full of uncertainty. But from that uncertainty can come creative approaches to defining our roles. It is encouraging that nurses are empowering themselves. A sign of self-directed growth from within supports the fact that nursing is moving away from an occupational to a professional group.

Levels of academic preparation

Fortunately, the issue of clinical nurse specialism has recently been clarified (UKCC, 1994). This will undoubtedly reduce the confusion in terminology and jargon used to date. More importantly, it will also provide a professional framework for practitioners wishing to pursue 'specialist' status. It is important to note that the term 'specialist' is not synonymous with its US counterpart. American specialist nurses are prepared to a Masters level of academic attainment. In the UK, it is advanced nurse practitioners who are formally required to achieve Masters level preparation.

The criteria for specialist practice preparation were initially set out by the UKCC (1986) in the document *Project 2000: A New Preparation for Practice*, the transition period for which ended in October 1998. Criteria for specialist practitioner programmes from that date state that academic study should be no less than first degree level and that the length of the programme must be no less than one academic year.

Clarification as to the level of academic preparation can only serve to further develop the level of professionalism in nursing. The framework ensures practitioners are aware of the 'credentials' of nurse specialists.

Scope of professional practice

The scope of specialist practice within the primary care setting has been identified by Wallace and Gough (1995) (see Box 11.2).

Box 11.2
Scope of specialist practice within primary care

■ General practice nursing
■ Community mental health nursing
■ Community mental handicap nursing
■ Community children's nursing
■ Health visiting
■ Occupational health nursing
■ District nursing
■ School nursing

However, areas of specialist practice within non-primary health care settings have not been defined. Indeed the council (UKCC, 1994) do not intend to describe specific areas. Leaving the playing field open like this can only be good for developing professional specialist nursing practice. Consumerist philosophy dictates that all services should be consumer-led. The health service is no exception. The consumer-led philosophy has been government policy in the post-Griffiths era (Griffiths, 1992). As a profession, we now have the flexibility to develop specialist programmes reflecting public demand and the need to fulfil professional growth within the dynamic environment of health care practice.

According to the RCN (1987), the driving forces for specialism are a result of the following factors:

'the need for a more effective use of manpower; the changing sociological, cultural and economic factors affecting health care; advances and changes in medical practice; specific needs of a population; developing national priorities in health care.'

(RCN 1988, p. 5)

Advancing nursing practice

In the old days, 'speciality status' often became a right, from attendance on short courses, or from working in an area, or with a client group other than 'general ward work'. This had the potential for specialists to appear 'precious' or self-important. It also led 'non-specialists' to be suspicious of their counterpart's credentials. This often resulted in a lack of respect. Benner (1984) suggested that one of the criteria for an expert is that they are revered as a learned person by others from within the same profession.

The opportunity for specialist practice is open to all areas where nurses interact with clients. The criteria have been stated and an apparent limitless window of opportunity exists. According to Styles (1989), the greatest challenge in the study of contemporary nursing specialisation is the identification of the specialities themselves. This leads one to question what areas warrant specialisation, and what potential frameworks exist. An example of such a framework was put forward by Styles in 1989, and can be seen in Table 11.2.

Table 11.2
A framework of specialisms (Styles, 1989) (Reprinted with permission from Margretta Styles. On Specialization in Nursing: Toward a New Empowerment, © 1989 American Nurses Publishing, American Nurses Foundation/ American Nurses Association, Washington DC 20024–2571)

Diseases/pathology	Oncology, diabetes, developmental disabilities, burns and trauma
Systems	Cardiovascular, pulmonary, neurological, renal
Ages	Paediatric: infant, child, adolescent Adult: maternity, geriatrics, etc.
Acuity	Emergency care, critical care, chronic illness, primary care
Settings	Community, school
Technologies/therapies	Anaesthesia, I.V. therapy
Functions or roles	Administration, teaching

The criteria in Table 11.2 were endorsed by the ICN (1992) and are based on the work of Styles (1989) (see Box 11.3). The ICN proposed that specialities develop along the curricula for general practice. Those outlined included medicine/surgery, maternity, paediatrics, mental health, geriatric and public health.

Box 11.3
Criteria for approval of specialities (ICN, 1992)

1. The speciality defines itself as nursing and subscribes to the overall purpose, functions and ethics of nursing.
2. The speciality practice is sufficiently complex and advanced that it is beyond the scope of general nursing practice.
3. There is both demand and need for the speciality service.
4. The focus of the speciality is a defined population that demonstrates recurrent problems and phenomena that lie within the discipline and practice of nursing.
5. The speciality practice is based on a core body of nursing knowledge which is continually being expanded and refined by research. Mechanisms exist for supporting, reviewing and disseminating research.

6. The speciality has established educational and practice standards which are congruent with those of the profession and are set by a recognised nursing body/ies.
7. The speciality adheres to the licensure/registration requirements for the general nurse.
8. Speciality expertise is obtained through a professionally approved advanced education programme which leads to a recognised qualification. The educational programme preparing the specialist is administered by a nurse.
9. The speciality has a credentialing process determined by the profession or in accordance with national practice for other professions. Sufficient human and financial resources are available to support this process.
10. Practitioners are organised and represented within a speciality association or a branch of the national nurses' association.

Specialism versus generalism

The field of rehabilitation nursing spans a multitude of clinical areas along life's continuum. The various fields are too numerous to list here. It is, however, pertinent to note that 'rehabilitation' occurs in areas by degrees. These include areas that are:

- rehabilitation specific, i.e. specialist rehabilitation hospitals and units,
- rehabilitation focused, i.e., utilise large components of rehabilitation principles, and
- rehabilitation 'in development', i.e. incorporate facets of rehabilitation principles.

Rehabilitation principles should be promoted in all care environments. It is doubtful that any rehabilitation nurse would argue that rehabilitation should occur in all stages of a client's or outpatient environment. Rehabilitation nurses have strong philosophical values that are reflected in clinical practice. Such philosophical values are outlined in Box 11.4.

Box 11.4
RCN standards of care (RNF, 1994, with permission)

1. They should be building on their knowledge base and participating in research relevant to rehabilitation.
2. Rehabilitation should commence at the onset of illness.
3. An interdisciplinary approach is essential if rehabilitation based on goal planning is to achieve the best outcome for client and family.
4. Effectiveness and continuity in rehabilitation can only be achieved through the provision of a 24 hour-a-day/7 day-a-week interdisciplinary service.
5. Clients are people with individual personalities and needs.

6. They have a role to play in educating nurses and other professionals in rehabilitation.
7. Communication is vital to the rehabilitation process.
8. Clients have a right to privacy, dignity and have the right to say 'no'.
9. Recreation, leisure and social interaction are important aspects of rehabilitation.
10. Clients are entitled to have a high standard of care from a named registered nurse and therapists.
11. A framework is needed to assess, plan and evaluate care which should be developed in partnership with client and family.
12. A health promotion focus is necessary to enable clients to concentrate on health and wellness rather than on disability and illness.
13. Education should be ongoing and must cater for the specialist needs of rehabilitation for staff, clients and relatives.

Rehabilitation nurse specialist

The above values reflect the unique beliefs about the rights of rehabilitation clients. Such beliefs are deeply grounded in rehabilitation nursing practice. One could argue that the approach taken by rehabilitation nurses is different from general nurses of the 'acute mind set'. This is because rehabilitation nurses view clients from a different perspective. They analyse clients from a multidimensional holistic angle, using a problem-solving approach. They interact with clients and involve them in their care, putting them at the centre of the care planning process. Rehabilitation nurses aim to enable clients to negotiate their own stepping stones to achieve their ultimate rehabilitation goals (within their own limitations). This approach is at the centre of rehabilitation nursing practice and reflects the true value of rehabilitation nursing. The cost-effectiveness of rehabilitation (and hence rehabilitation nursing) has been questioned (McKenna et al., 1992). Evidence of the effectiveness of rehabilitation, such as the positive outcomes from stroke units, has been reported (Langhorne, 1993). The effectiveness of the specialist nurse (including the rehabilitation nurse specialist) has also been questioned. One of the difficulties the profession has faced is that nursing outcomes are often described as intangible. This therefore makes them difficult to measure. Wilson-Barnet and Beech (1994) reported that the role of the nurse specialist is measurable, and indeed cost-effective.

I would concur with the sentiment that:

'. . . there is a need for future research efforts to combine these (evaluation) methods, establish stronger relationships, and *refine outcome and cost analysis measures; only then will the true value of the specialist nurse be truly recognised.'*

(Wilson-Barnet and Beech, 1994)

Henderson (1980) has argued that nurses are rehabilitators par excellence. This has been challenged by others (Gibbons, 1993; Myco, 1984; O'Connor, 1993). Myco (1984) suggested that *rehabilitators par excellence* would not be realised until nurses develop the confidence, through the acquisition of appropriate knowledge and skill, to structure a specific role in stroke client care. A decade later, this 'appropriate knowledge' and skill does appear to be being gained. However, this is occurring at a time when the process of rehabilitation is being eroded. This appears to be most prevalent in those environments which were the last to develop a true rehabilitation ethos; namely acute hospital wards. With the seemingly never ending 'efficiency improvements' and 'cost-containment exercises' there is potential for rehabilitation to be seriously affected. Clients are at risk of not achieving their ultimate rehabilitation goals, which may be within their limits but out of the limits of the NHS's 'limited resources'. The constant squeezing of resources that the health service is experiencing today, adopting short-term financial outlooks, is compromising the beliefs and values that rehabilitation nurses hold so close to their hearts. The value of rehabilitation must be exhibited by undertaking further research and refining rehabilitation nursing outcomes. A variety of opportunities are available from both quantitative and qualitative methods.

It could be argued that there are two different and distinct environs in which rehabilitation nursing takes place, (excluding the primary health care settings). One is the 'ring fenced' establishment, used specifically for rehabilitation clients. Such areas generally include rehabilitation-specific units and centres. The second area is rehabilitation wards and 'units' which are often an intrinsic part of district general hospitals (DGHs). These rehabilitation beds tend not to be ring-fenced. From personal experience and reports from colleagues they often tend to be 'elderly' areas. These rehabilitation units appear to be the first to deal with patients who have fallen between health and social care. These are individuals who often require semi-continuing care or are awaiting nursing or rest-home placement. This compounds the problem for nurses who have to wear two hats: 'passive carer', giving total nursing care, and rehabilitation nurse, striving to uphold an important and unique set of beliefs and values. Such a conflict has the potential to be stressful for all staff.

One could argue that as a result of the varying culture and, philosophies, there are two types of rehabilitation nurse. The first type is the one in a 'genuine rehabilitation setting'. The second is the one who works in a 'semi-rehabilitation setting'. The latter may end up feeling like a 'second cousin' to a 'true' rehabilitation nurse.

There may be many reasons for this. One reason may be that rehabilitation centres have the power to control admission to their units. Secondly, it is possible that many such centres have age-related admission criteria. This has many implications, not least the reflection of societal prejudices discriminating against older people. Thirdly, it would appear that many DGH rehabilitation wards are for older people. This is because during the 1980s, DGHs closed continuing care facilities, and many nurses found themselves 'drifting' into the subsequently developed 'rehabilitation units', most of which were rehabilitation units only in name. In many areas this happened without staff being adequately prepared for the 'brave new world' they were to experience, not to mention what was expected of them.

Traditional elderly care environments were primarily concerned with 'caring for' and not 'caring about' clients. In this model, the client played the role of a grateful and passive recipient of care. Patients were done 'to' and 'for' and seldom 'with'. These practices are still observable in such environments today. The area of gerontology and hence elderly rehabilitation is the largest growing area within the health care system (DoH, 1991). The demand for elderly rehabilitation services is expected to increase significantly towards the millennium and beyond. Advances in health care science are also resulting in an increased demand for 'non-elderly' rehabilitative services. After years of being a 'Cinderella service', rehabilitation is becoming a high priority area. This is recognised by the DoH who, in collaboration with the RCN in 1997, set up a task force to look into the role of the rehabilitation nurse.

As stated previously, rehabilitation is an all-encompassing discipline transcending the continuum of life. For this reason, specialism in rehabilitation nursing should adopt a generalist approach. The criteria for rehabilitation courses aims to provide a 'common theoretical base'. This is essential to underpin all rehabilitation nursing practice. It is such a common theoretical base which should be universal amongst rehabilitation nurses. It would seem logical for rehabilitation courses to operate a 'core and cluster' system. This would mean the major course content having a generalist rehabilitation content (core) and additional condition-specific elements (cluster), i.e. stroke, Parkinson's, head injury, respiratory, and so on.

According to Davis (1996), rehabilitation should be developed around the beliefs outlined in Box 11.5.

Box 11.5

Beliefs around which rehabilitation should be developed (Davis, 1996, with permission)

- Beliefs about rehabilitation
- Beliefs about disabled individuals
- Beliefs about professional practice and
- Beliefs about education

Beliefs about rehabilitation need to be person-centred. According to Armentrout (1993), nurses are in a strategic position to plan rehabilitation goals in partnership with the disabled person (and where appropriate, their family/carer). The nurse is part of the rehabilitation team. One of the central philosophies to rehabilitation nursing (RCN, 1994) is related to teamwork and effective interdisciplinary communication.

For the rehabilitation nurse, the emphasis is on the *person* who is disabled (not the *disabled* person). It is all about putting the person first and recognising their rights. Rehabilitation nurses are empathic. This is evident by the fact that practice is moving towards a client focus and away from a professional or hospital focus. Central to rehabilitation nursing is having the ability to give unconditional positive regard. This is why rehabilitation nurses find prejudices so hard to swallow.

Professional practice should focus on enabling, facilitating and empowering a person who is disabled, to achieve a good quality of life. The rehabilitation nurse is a client's support mechanism and (at times) an advocate. The professional rehabilitation nurse specialist should have the knowledge skills and competencies to give their best for a disabled person. Such knowledge, skills and competencies should have a common theoretical base whether one is caring about an elderly person recovering from a stroke or a young person who has sustained a head injury.

The rehabilitation nurse specialist should develop a comprehensive research-based knowledge of rehabilitation, and strive to give care that is best practice. As the rehabilitation nurse specialist is part of a multidisciplinary team, mutual respect of each profession, their roles, responsibilities and areas of overlap is essential. The scope to improve knowledge through interprofessional teaching and ultimately formalised training has been reported (Walker, 1995a, 1995b). However, difficulty associated with integrated training has been reported (Walker, 1995b). With the current evolutionary state of the National Health Service, the time is ripe for opportunities in enhancing the role of the rehabilitation nurse. As professionals, we owe it to ourselves and our clients to grasp such opportunities.

Conclusion

Rehabilitation deals with people who have multiple needs (Diller, 1990) and demonstrates the breadth and complexity of the speciality (Melvin, 1989). It is a subject which is far greater than the sum of its constituent parts. If rehabilitation nurses are going to give an optimal service to people who are disabled, surely they need to have a comprehensive education and adequate preparation via a common theoretical base. Such extensive preparation gives the rehabilitation nurse specialist the opportunity to draw on valuable unique experiences, upon which to reflect when presented with rehabilitation nursing problems. To receive preparation in only a part of rehabilitation can only disadvantage the nurse and (potentially) the client. Fragmentation of rehabilitation nurse specialist training also has the potential to reduce the validity of it being viewed as a true specialism.

References

Appel, A.L., Malcolm, p.A. & Nahas. V (1996) Nursing specialisation in New South Wales, Australia. *Clinical Nurse Specialist*, **10**, 76–81.

Appel, A. L., Malcolm, P. A. & Nahcas, V. (1996) Nursing specialisation in New South Wales, Australia. *Clinical Nurse Specialist*, **10**, 76–81.

Armentrout, G. A. (1993) Comparison of the Medical Model and the Wellness Model: The Importance of Knowing the Difference. *Holistic Nursing Practice*, **7**, 57–62.

Benner, P. (1984) *From Novice to Expert Professional*. California: Addison-Wesley.

Berne, E. (1984) *What Do You Say After You Say Hello?* London: Corgi.

Buchanan, L. C. (1992) Rehabilitation clinical nurse specialist: evaluation of the role in a home health care setting. *Holistic Nursing Practice*, **6**, 42–50.

Butterworth, T. (1994) Preparing to take on clinical supervision. *Nursing Standard*, **8**, 32–34.

Davis, S. M. (1996) *Studies in Rehabilitation; Student Handbook*. Oxford: School of Health Care, Oxford Brookes University.

Diller, L. (1990) Fostering the interdisciplinary team, fostering research in a society in transition. *Archives of Physical and Medical Rehabilitation*, **71**, 275–278.

Department of Health. (1991) *The Health of the Nation*. London: HMSO.

Elliott, P. (1997) A Community Hospital Perspective on Advanced Nursing Practice. In *Advanced Nursing Practice*, ed. Rolfe, G. & Fulbrooke. P, p. 168. Oxford: Butterworth Heinemann.

Gibbons, B. (1993) Implications for nurses in the management of stroke rehabilitation: a review of the literature. *International Journal of Nursing Studies*, **30**, 133–141.

Girard, N. (1987) In *The Clinical Nurse Specialist; Perspectives on Practice*. New York: John Wiley.

Griffiths, R. (1992) *The N. H.· S. Management Enquiry. Working for Patients*. London: HMSO.

Habel, M. (1993) Rehabilitation nursing practice. In *The Speciality Practice of Rehabilitation Nursing: A Core Curriculum*, 3rd edn, ed. McCourt, A. E., Skokie I., I.: Rehabilitation Nursing Foundation of the Association of Rehabilitation Nurses.

Hamric & Spross, (1989) *The Clinical Nurse Specialist in Theory and Practice*, 2nd edn. Philadelphia: W. B. Saunders Co.

Henderson, V. (1980) Preserving the Essence of Nursing in a Technological Age. *Journal of Advanced Nursing Studies*, **5**, 245–260.

Hoeffer, B. & Murphy, S. A. (1984) Issues in *Professional Nursing*: Specialisation in Nursing Practice, pp. 1–13. Washington DC: American Nurses Association.

Hunt, G. & Wainwright, P. (1994) *Expanding the Role of the Nurse: The Scope of Professional Practice*. London: Blackwell Scientific Publications, 101–112.

International Council of Nurses. (1992) *Guidelines on Specialisation in Nursing*. Geneva, Switzerland: International Council of Nurses.

Langhorne, P. et al. (1993) Do Stroke Units Save Lives? *The Lancet*, **342**, 395–398.

Lunt, p. (1995) The hands-on specialist nurse in renal care. *Professional Nurse*, **11**, 17–19.

McKenna, M., Maynard, A., Wright. K, et al. (1992) Is rehabilitation cost effective? (Discussion Paper 101). York: University of York, Centre for Heath Economics.

Melvin, J. L. (1989) Status Report of Interdisciplinary Medical Rehabilitation. *Archives of Physical Medicine and Rehabilitation*, **70**, 273–277.

Miller, S. (1995) The clinical nurse specialist: a way forward: *Journal of Advanced Nursing Practice*, **22**, 494–501.

Myco, F. (1984) Stroke and its rehabilitation: the

perceived role of the nurse in the medical and nursing literature. *Journal of Advanced Nursing*, **9**, 429–439.

Nash, A. (1993) A stressful role. *Nursing Times*, **89**, 50–51.

O'Connor, S. (1993) Nursing and rehabilitation: the interventions of nurses in stroke patient care. *Journal of Clinical Nursing*, **2**, 29–34.

O'Hanlon, M. & Gibbon, S. (1996) Advanced practice. *Nursing Management*, **2**, 12–13.

Rehabilitation Nurses Forum. (1994) To be supplied.

Royal College of Nursing (1988) *Specialities in Nursing*. London: Royal College of Nursing.

Royal College of Nursing. (1994) *Standards of Care: Rehabilitation Nursing*. London: Royal College of Nursing.

Ryan, S. (1996) Defining the role of the specialist nurse. *Nursing Standard*, **10**, 27–29.

Storr, G. (1988) The clinical nurse specialist: from the outside looking in. *Journal of Advanced Nursing* **13**, 265–272.

Styles, M. (1989) *On Specialization in Nursing: Toward a New Empowerment*. Washington: American Nurses Foundation.

United Kingdom Central Council (1986) *Project 2000; A Preparation for Practice*. London: United Kingdom Central Council.

United Kingdom Central Council (1994) *The Future of Professional Practice – the Council's Standards for Education and Practice Following Registration*. London: United Kingdom Central Council for Nursing, Midwifery and Health Visiting.

Vitello-Ciccui, J. (1984) Excellence in critical care. Educating the clinical specialist. *Critical Care Quarterly*, **7**, 26–32.

Walker, G. (1995a) Editorial. *British Journal of Therapy and Rehabilitation*, **2**, 59–60.

Walker, A. (1995b) Multidisciplinary education in the health care profession. *British Journal of Therapy and Rehabilitation*, **2**, 5–6.

Wallace, M. & Gough, P. (1995) The U.K.C.C.'s criteria for specialist and advanced nursing practice. *British Journal of Nursing*, **4**, 939–944.

Wilson-Barnett, J. & Beech, S. (1994) Evaluating the clinical nurse specialist: a review. *International Journal of Nursing Studies*, **31**, 561–571.

12 The role of the generic worker

Lesley Crabtree

Key issues
- Role and purpose of the generic worker
- The argument supporting the role
- The argument challenging the role
- Controversy surrounding the development of the role for rehabilitation

Introduction

The concept of the generic worker role is both contemporary and controversial. Even within health care in the UK, there are many perceptions of the generic worker where the differences centre on who they are and what they do. A professional generic worker role would seem to have a particular place in meeting the rehabilitation needs of clients of all ages, and yet its emergence and development remain confusing and uncertain. This chapter considers why nurses or any other health care professionals would argue for the role of the generic worker in rehabilitation.

There are a range of terms used to describe various generic roles which equally may be termed generic workers. These are represented in Box 12.1.

Box 12.1
Different terms used for generic worker

> **Registered professional**
> Generic nurse
> Generic role
> Generic (professional) carer
> Generic therapist
>
> **Non-professional**
> Generic assistant
> Generic carer
> Generic support worker
> Generic worker

Role and purpose of the generic worker

A review of the available published literature reveals a dearth of discussion about the role of a generic professional worker with specialist skills and cross-professional and interdisciplinary knowledge. Such a generic worker for rehabilitation could have rehabilitation skills using knowledge that is currently placed within nursing, physiotherapy and occupational therapy. Likewise, there is a dearth of literature representing the generic worker as a non-professional employed for the purpose of assisting members of the multiprofessional team. Instead, discussion about the non-professional generic worker focuses on a role that can be supervised by nurses (Anderson, 1997; Leifer, 1996; University of Manchester Health Services Management Unit, 1996)

Other perspectives view the generic worker as someone who has received a generalist nurse education or training to equip them with a broad range of skills and attributes that will address the nursing needs of a wide variety of client groups. This was certainly the model that was thought to be emerging within nursing as the debate around Project 2000 developed in the mid 1980s. The concept of the generic nurse or 'nurse of all trades' was envisaged as (Kratz 1985), arising from all student nurses receiving a common foundation element of the nursing course. More recently in the 1990s, the generic registered nurse has been contemplated by the proposed merging of the four main branches of nursing (adult, paediatric, mental health and learning disabilities). Rowden (1993) suggests that such a practitioner could meet the many common needs of clients in all care settings in a flexible manner. He proposes a common 3-year course which would lead to registration. This could then be progressed by specialist post-basic programmes to diploma or degree level (Rowden, 1993). This is the approach adopted in many other countries, and reflects the perceived need for a multi-skilled flexible practitioner. While there is some resistance or caution about this idea (Mangan, 1993; Thomas, 1993), it offers the opportunity to prepare registered generic nurses with rehabilitative skills that would meet common needs in the broad range of care settings, but who can go on to specialise and gain further post-registration qualifications.

An alternative perspective envisages the generic worker as offering nurses the opportunity to extend their practice and responsibilities. To date, this debate takes two forms. The first considers nurses expanding their role, primarily into areas traditionally perceived as medical. This is a concept not fully supported by many nurses. The second considers the removal or merging of professional boundaries (Dyson, 1992). For example, the merging of district nurses and health visitors to offer a multiprofessional role in the community, so helping to remove current barriers to continuity of care. Already, certain components of community courses are shared by the different community disciplines, for example, district nurses, health visitors, school nurses and practice nurses. If these were extended, they could be organised to offer multiple qualifications to a single individual nurse, as does occur in some cases.

Within the debate about rehabilitative care, it is not the generic nature of a nurse's role that is contemplated. The creation of a new rehabilitation professional, called the generic worker, is envisaged to incorporate the skills of a wider range of disciplines such as nursing, physiotherapy, occupational therapy, speech therapy and complementary medicine. This offers a radical review of the person who works alongside the client during rehabilitative care.

The proposal for a multiprofessional generic worker was a focus within the 1996 report by the University of Manchester, Health Services Management Unit, which looked at the future health care workforce of the UK. This report aimed to examine and match future workforce needs to the contemporary changes occurring within health care provision and services, such as the move towards greater developments within primary care. The authors identified a drive within the NHS for increased flexibility, and argued for the emergence of a spectrum of roles that would break down the current demarcation between different professional disciplines and support workers. The spectrum could develop, they suggest, by the bridging of current roles with the introduction of the generic worker, who they termed the 'generic professional carer'. This would require that future educational courses could deliver the broader based 'generic carer' rather than a range of single professions. On leaving a common core programme, generic carers would be trained to a basic level of understanding of client needs in particular service areas identified as primary care, mental health, and general and acute hospitals. It is suggested that this would free up the specialist, for example, nurse, doctor or therapist, allowing them to clearly define and utilise their specific training and expertise, and focus on skilled activities such as assessment and planning of care along with evaluation. The 'generic carer' would carry out and coordinate most of this planned care. In some ways, this concept seems to make sense, since it could be argued that it is unrealistic to expect new health care employees to specialise at a very early stage. Choices made later would surely be linked to a more certain knowledge base (Rowden, 1993). Significantly, they also suggest that a staff skill-mix can be designed to meet client need. The report's authors believe that the evidence for an extension of the support workforce is compelling. While they do not suggest that an increase in the proportion of 'generic carers' would lead to a reduction in the number of specialist professionals, it would seem that this would be a natural consequence. This report only focused upon specific areas such as primary care, mental health and general and acute hospitals. It did not in fact consider specific client groups such as those needing rehabilitation. However, it is conceivable that the role of the 'generic carer' could be extended to encompass the needs of this care group. Additionally, the report did not give consideration to the specialised skills currently offered by experienced nurses with speciality expertise such as those found in some areas of rehabilitation.

Since the University of Manchester report, the debate continues to encompass a diversity of generic worker models and there is no recognised education or training for the role, as yet. This continues to be determined at a local level, and is most likely to involve working to gain a National Vocational qualification. While no nationally recognised and accredited role exists, the inconsistency and uncertainty of what is desired persists.

Within rehabilitation, where professionals are now recognising that an understanding of each other's skills and knowledge best serves the needs of disabled people, there is the opportunity to take the lead and define and develop the generic worker role. This could arise from a consensus which considers the arguments both to support and challenge the development of a new registered practitioner whose work would arise from consultation with the multiprofessional team. However, if there is further delay, this may not be an option as the driving forces for a generic worker role are gaining momentum.

The argument supporting the role

The forces driving the emergence of the generic worker may take a number of perspectives. From the perspective of the client with rehabilitation needs, the ideology is that the generic worker represents someone who has the diverse and varied skills of at least the nurse and therapists. This overcomes the client's dilemma of who to call on for help, because the role offers someone with an integrated approach who readily reinforces the aims of care and who, in the hospital setting, is available over a 24-hour period. This means that, regardless of time, as clients need professional help, there is someone available offering appropriate care. This removes the disruption so often experienced by clients when the particular specialist, nurse or therapist, is not available or not on duty. It moves towards the notion of seamless care advocated for effective health and social care (The NHS and Community Care Act 1993), and means that as need arises, it may be met. It also helps to avoid the confusion between professionals about who is providing care, or duplication of services and inefficient use of client and staff time.

As health care provision is increasingly provided in the community, a model that determines the direction of specialist nursing will benefit both clients (Wade and Moyer, 1989) and nurses (Haste and MacDonald, 1992). The issue for the generic worker role is how to develop the role alongside a specialised nursing service that meets the needs of clients. As Layzell and McCarthy (1993) say:

'It is vital to distinguish between creating direct-care specialist posts or teams and employing individual nurses with specialised knowledge and skills to act as a resource to existing staff.'

The future rehabilitative service must enable the development of roles, including nursing and the generic worker, so that comprehensive and specialist provision is available to clients wherever they need it.

An additional perspective is the apparently inevitable development of a flexible workforce of multi-skilled practitioners. If education and training integrates current professional approaches to care, and staff qualify with a generic range of skills, then there will be improved understanding about how to provide care for clients with a broad range of problems.

From an economic and financial perspective, the generic worker role could reduce staffing costs by performing much of the work normally delivered by a range of professionals. This not only reduces the number of specialist professionals required but ensures, as already suggested, continuity of care. This notion is supported by Scullion (1997) who suggests that:

> 'capturing and encouraging the features of optimal rehabilitation practice, characterised by blending professional roles according to patients, holds out great potential.'

This view is supported by Castledine (1994) who acknowledges that 'no single profession is likely to be capable of meeting the consumers' needs alone'.

From a managerial perspective there is no doubt that such a development would be attractive. If it was to lead to a more efficient use and spread of skills, so as to enhance the continuity and perhaps quality of care for clients so speeding up their recovery, then it could be seen as both a cost-efficient and effective move. Similarly, if there was the possibility that it would widen the opportunities for the recruitment of staff, then it could be seen as necessary.

The argument challenging the role

The responses that counter the proposal for a generic worker role also take a number of perspectives. From a client's perspective, the argument against the generic worker is that the care delivered would not be as expert as that they would receive from the specialist professional. The proposal for a single individual to become adequately proficient in the variety of skills and knowledge attributed to different professions is unrealistic. Large areas of practice are unique to the individual professions and it would be unworkable to be offering a role that is all to everyone. The skills of a broad-based generic worker would be so diluted as to leave them unable even to maintain standards. They would be unable to keep pace or up-to-date with the broader field and rapid changes in health care, and this could also impact detrimentally on standards of care. This argument could be offset by the suggestion that by enabling the specialists to focus and concentrate on their area of interest, they are in fact in a more beneficial position to maintain and develop their expertise.

An ongoing criticism of health service provision has been the lack of coordination and integration of care delivered to individuals. It is difficult to foresee how the communication difficulties presently acknowledged within multiprofessional teams could be overcome since the generic worker will still need to liaise with all the team members. Therefore all issues of availability, improved quality of service and uncertainty about each other's roles could still be irreconcilable. It is unlikely that the current difficulties and restrictions experienced in trying to coordinate and meet, for example, to arrange a prompt case conference or general team meeting, will be removed. The generic worker may also find themselves in a compromised position. If their role is to coordinate and carry out care, as well as support and reinforce actions determined by other team members, then they themselves, as the direct client carer, may both feel and be de-skilled. This would simply be a repetition of the position of current support workers.

Nurses may fear that with the introduction of the generic worker, their contact with clients would diminish, hence the effectiveness of client care and their own professional identity would be compromised. One view has been (Editorial, 1996) that the generic worker, as proposed by the University of Manchester report (1996), would simply reflect the core of the existing nurses' role. This response, however, would seem to assume that nurses currently have the skills and knowledge to meet most rehabilitative needs of their clients. It is perhaps naive, since currently nurses do not adequately meet the rehabilitative needs of many clients. In a similar way, it seems that occupational therapists believe that they respond to a wide range of client needs and conditions, providing rehabilitation that minimizes disability and impairment as well as giving preventative advice (Crawford-White, 1996). As with nurses, their stance is to retain and nurture their professional identity because large areas of practice are unique to that individual profession.

While the development of a generic worker may be seen as a more effective and efficient way of delivering care, there is also the possibility that it could be used as an exercise to substitute qualified staff and dilute skills, so acting as a cost-cutting initiative. There is also a fear that the new role could be exploited to reduce the establishment of qualified nursing staff. This would depend upon the way or ways in which the generic worker was developed. However, managers would be wise to consider and take account of the number of studies that have demonstrated that a higher skill-mix leads ultimately to more effective and efficient care, leading to better outcomes.

The controversy surrounding the development of the role for rehabilitation

Perhaps one of the most significant challenges to the successful implementation of the role of the generic worker is the involvement of all the professional groups within rehabilitation. At the local level, the effectiveness of interdisciplinary working has limitations. This includes the barriers to effective teamworking, the failure to agree common aims, professional tribalism and structural and organisational deficits (ENB, 1997). The fear of each, that their particular professional identity may risk being lost, may well lead to considerable resistance. This concern is perhaps not unreasonable given the historical development of the different professions. Contemporary practice and experience suggests that there remains strong rivalry between professions, despite efforts to work towards interdisciplinary working. Thus, the belief that large areas of practice are unique to individual professions would seem to question the feasibility of introducing a generic worker. This view has added weight if it is believed that a generic worker 'cannot be all to everyone'. However, this may be unjustified since the importance of each profession would still seem to be key. This would very much depend upon the way the role of the generic worker was introduced and the way that the individual professional disciplines worked and developed with them.

Shared or multi- and interdisciplinary education is already gaining momentum, but uncertainty remains about how radical curriculum development should be, and whether this includes a common core curriculum for all health care roles with the earliest exit point being for the generic worker.

The more the development of the generic worker role is pursued, the more questions arise that need to be answered.

Conclusion

The work of defining the generic worker role should take account of the needs of both client and carer and should therefore involve clients and carers. Rehabilitation needs arise for people remaining at home, in the hospital setting and in the community again, post-discharge. The development of roles needs to acknowledge this.

In order to further the potential of nursing for meeting the rehabilitation needs of clients, nurses should take the lead in developing the generic worker role. This will include deciding:

- what specific place nurses have in meeting clients' needs wherever they are
- how the generic worker relates to nurses
- where primary responsibility for direct care is placed.

All the professionals who have an interest in the generic worker role should work together. They would need to:

- determine the authority of the generic worker and to whom they are professionally accountable

- agree on the planning and implementation of the new role
- decide about education and training that enables the development of the generic worker role and the specialisation of each of the professions
- determine the professional criteria for the generic worker, how they become a registered practitioner and the form of regulatory body.

Questions for discussion

- What would the role of generic worker be in your area?
- What are barriers to this role and how could they be overcome?
- What would the advantages be?
- What are the implications for professionals?

Acknowledgements

I would like to thank Sian Wade for her help and support during the preparation of this chapter.

References

Anderson, L. (1997) The role and resources required for the introduction of generic ward assistants using GRASP systems workload methodology: a quantitative study. *Journal of Nursing Management*, **5**, 11–17.

Castledine, G. (1994) The role of nurses in the 21st Century. *British Journal of Nursing*, **3**, 621–622.

Crawford-White, J. (1996) Are primary health care occupational therapists specialists or generalists? *British Journal of Therapy and Rehabilitation*, **3**, 373–379.

Dyson, R. (1992) *Changing Labour Utilisation in the NHS Trusts*. London: NHS Management Executive.

Editorial. (1996) Pandora's box of tricks. *Nursing Times*, **92**, 3.

Nolan, M. R., Booth, A. & Nolan, J. (1997) Preparation for multi-professional/multi-agency health care practice: the nursing contribution to rehabilitation within the multi-disciplinary team. A literature review and curriculum analysis. *Research Highlights 28*. London: English National Board.

Haste, F. H. & MacDonald, L. D. (1992) The role of the specialist in community nursing: perceptions of specialist and district nurses. *International Journal of Nursing Studies*, **29**, 37–47.

Kratz, C. (1985) Project 2000: nurse of all trades? . . . a generic nurse. *Nursing Times*, **81**, 32–33.

Layzell, S. & McCarthy, M. (1993) Specialist or generic community nursing care for HIV/AIDs patients? *Journal of Advanced Nursing*, **18**, 531–537.

Leifer, D. (1996) Public outcry greets plans for 'generic worker' [news] *Nursing Standard*, **10**, 12.

Mangan, P. (1993) A dream ticket? . . . the pros and cons of the generic nurse. *Nursing Times*, **89**, 26–28.

Rowden, R. (1993) Breaking the mould. *Nursing Times*, **89**, 29–30.

Scullion, P. (1997) Rehabilitation nurses: are they coming of age? *British Journal of Therapy and Rehabilitation*, 4, 580–581.

Thomas, B. (1993) A dilution of skills . . . the generic nurse. *Nursing Times*, **89**, 30–31.

University of Manchester Health Services Management Unit. (1996) The future health care workforce. *The Steering Group Report*. Manchester: University of Manchester Health Services Management Unit.

Wade, B. & Moyer, A. (1989) An evaluation of clinical nurse specialists: implications for education and organisation of care. *Senior Nurse*, 9, 1–16.

13 Setting priorities in research

Stephen O'Connor

Key issues
- Rehabilitation nursing and a research agenda
- Research methods for rehabilitation nursing

Introduction

Rehabilitation nursing is a relatively new speciality within the nursing field. Although recognised early in the USA, in the UK, the specialist contribution of nurses to the rehabilitation process has been limited. This situation of limited understanding still exists today in some circles, for example, Worlow et al (1997) limit their vision of the input of the nurse in the multidisciplinary team to the revision of basic needs, daily assessment, the prevention of complications and support for relatives. This is, however, an improvement on earlier expectations that the nurse's role is to support the therapist and maintain the ward environment (Feigenson, 1981). This chapter has therefore two objectives, first, to discuss an agenda for research within rehabilitation nursing and secondly, to outline the appropriateness of different research approaches to rehabilitation nursing.

Rehabilitation nursing and a research agenda

The youthful nature of rehabilitation nursing has resulted in the understandable concentration of researchers on the role of the nurse (Gibbons 1992; O'Connor 1993; Waters 1996). The focus of the 1997 RCN Rehabilitation Conference on rehabilitation as a philosophy of care simply reinforces this issue. The validity of such studies is unquestionable, as a clear picture of the nature of the nursing interventions in rehabilitation is essential, but as such studies and discussions denote, consensus is emerging. The time is now to move on to address the validity of these particular nursing interventions and their importance on the clients' outcomes. Research in the sphere of rehabilitation nursing can therefore be seen to have two specific areas to address. First, the broad question of the value of the nurses' contribution to the rehabilitation process, and secondly, the value of the individual aspects of the nurses' contribution.

The first of these spheres is the most difficult in terms of both the clarity of the question and the possibility of a practical research method. If the contribution of nursing practice to rehabilitation outcomes is to be identified, the first problem is the question of the identification of good practice. As can be seen, this brings back the problem outlined above as to the identification of the nature of the nursing interventions, which have to be identified before an area can be said to demonstrate them.

Given that such sites can be identified, the next problem is the issue of how to identify that the specialist nurse in such locations does actually improve the clients' outcomes. The ability to contrast the input of such nurses on client outcomes with that of non-specialist nurses is complicated by the impact of the nature of the location. Almost by definition, specialist nurses will work in special-ist areas, and as such, the enterprise is confused; what is being evaluated, the specialist nurses or the location? However, as it is assumed that specialist nursing such as rehabilitation, intensive care and paediatrics is only possible in specialist areas, then the problem is resolved. The question then becomes one of standardising of the other inputs, which in the case of rehabilitation implies the contri-bution of the therapists. What is then possible is a comparison between the outcomes of care delivered to a particular group of clients by specialist nurses in a specialist area, with that delivered to a similar client group by non-specialist nurses with as many other variables as possible remaining constant. Such studies will be able to determine the effect of specialist nursing on the outcomes of clients.

The importance of demonstrating that individual nursing inter-ventions are of value cannot be over-estimated. Once again, given that we know what these interventions are, the demonstration of their efficiency is a matter of methodology. However, a general dis-cussion of a programme of research for rehabilitation nursing is important as this would not only seek to validate the status quo in terms of practice, but also should be a way forward in terms of developments in practice.

The Rehabilitation Nurses Foundation (RNF), the research arm of the American rehabilitation organisation, the Association of Rehabilitation Nurses (ARN) has recently undertaken a major study to identify a prospective research programme for rehabilitation in the USA. The results of the study published by Gordon, Swain and Baster (1996) indicate that a consensus amongst rehabilitation nurses concerning research priorities does exist. Box 13.1 below lists the top items, these represent the items most consistently perceived as in need of increased knowledge in contextual and clinical spheres. The items identified under the heading of context relate directly to the theme discussed above. The broad theme of the impact of rehabilitation nursing is central, however other themes are per-ceived as essential; the impact of cost and skill-mix should also be noted.

Box 13.1
*Contextual and
clinical items deemed
in need of research
by the RNF*

Contextual items

1. Relationship of functional outcomes to type, intensity, and length of rehabilitation nursing services
2. The effect of changing healthcare priorities on the practice of rehabilitation nurses
3. Cost and contributions of rehabilitation nurses as a component of the rehabilitation process
4. Influence of rehabilitation nursing staff-mix on client outcomes

Clinical items

1. Interventions to support health-promoting behaviours in persons with disabilities
2. Effects of bladder management techniques on urinary tract infection, quality of life, and cost of care, in individuals with neurogenic bladder
3. Educational strategies to optimise client and family learning in rehabilitation
4. Therapeutics that enhance and maintain independence and self-care
5. Effects of care-giving on family members who care for individuals with chronic illness or disability in the home
6. Interventions to prevent physiological complications and secondary disabilities

Gordon, et al. 1996

The second feature of the research agenda, as stated earlier, is the impact of identifiable interventions perceived by rehabilitation nurses as their specific practice. The clinical section in Box 13.1 lists the top six items from a total of 25 considered worthy of further research. Within this list, three items are most noticeable as items that have been identified by all of the writers on the specialist interventions of the nurse in rehabilitation, i.e. bladder management, education strategies and psychological care. These three features are unsurprising, however items (1) and (4) are worthy of further note. The implications that nurses should concern themselves with interventions to support health-promoting behaviours in persons with a disability implies that the remit of the nurse is wider than that of caring in institutions. While such interventions are obviously part of the rehabilitation after a disabling incident, the implication is that the nurses' impact should be broader and longer-lasting. The second item of interest is that involved in item (5), that is the effects of care-giving on the care-givers. This sphere is associated with that discussed above, as it focuses on the longer-term effects of the nurses' input. The impact of long-term care-giving on care-givers should be seen as the mirror image of the ability of the disabled individual to maintain health-promoting behaviours. This relationship seems to reinforce the duality outlined by Orem (1991) of dependent care agency and self-care agency, highlighted in Chapter 1. The work of the RNF is of importance as it is broadly based and does have resonance with the situation, as identified by various writers in this country.

One further area of potential research is an assessment of the impact of the education of student and qualified nurses in the subject matter of rehabilitation. The recent English National Board (ENB) commissioned project to establish the nature and extent of rehabilitation nursing input in pre- and post-registration programmes, would seem to highlight both a general paucity of input and that there is a narrow approach taken (Nolan, Nolan and Mason, 1997). While such findings are of use to those who seek to increase the impact of rehabilitation nursing in such curricula, they do not come as any great surprise. The project does, however, raise two important issues; first, the role of the nurse in rehabilitation, and secondly, the place, impact and relative merit of rehabilitation nursing in pre- and post-registration education. The first of these two areas has already been addressed and the ENB project does not add more to the subject, merely reinforcing the perceptions of other writers. However, the second issue is much more relevant and needs to be addressed in a rational and constructive manner.

In the interests of clarity, a differentiation between pre- and post registration education needs to be made, as different outcomes of the educational process would seem to be expected. In the case of pre-registration, any curriculum can only be expected to cover the principles of rehabilitation nursing along with those associated skills that can be seen to be commensurate with the concept of competence required at that level. The function of research would seem, therefore, to be set at a level already undertaken by the ENB project, an assessment of what is in curricula. If a system does exist that can assess competency in enough detail to identify specific rehabilitation outcomes, then such could be addressed, but as yet, no such instrument has been published. In the case of post-registration education, the situation is different. Managers second staff onto post-registration courses with the specific aim of improving client care. This identifies a specific outcome that can be addressed in research terms. The task for rehabilitation nurse researchers is to develop sensitive instruments that can identify the impact of such education on client care. This will in turn feed back to the educationalists, who can then review the content of their courses so that there is a direct relationship between what the course delivers, what managers and practitioners deem as required, and most importantly, the impact on client care.

The above can only be seen as *an* agenda and not *the* agenda, and I am sure that other areas, perhaps more specific ones, come to mind. However, what has been outlined above is in line with developments both here in the UK and in the USA.

The last section of this chapter will identify some of the methods by which these questions may be addressed.

Research methods for rehabilitation nursing

In the space available, it is not possible to give detailed accounts of research strategies and methods; any of the many research textbooks will amply fulfil this role. What is possible is a general discussion on the ways rehabilitation research is addressed, and several factors that are important to, and impact upon, rehabilitation nurses within their practice areas regarding research.

The approach that researchers have taken to rehabilitation, and to a lesser extent rehabilitation nursing, has been divided between quantitative and qualitative approaches. Generally speaking, quantitative research has been centred upon the systematic collection of numerical data under what are deemed to be controlled conditions, and the resultant data being analysed through the use of accepted descriptive and inferential statistical techniques. Qualitative research is perceived to be an alternative form of research that does not rely on the collection of numerical data where quantification is seen as the goal. However, qualitative research is more than just data without numbers, it is a rich vein of information that gives insights, and attempts to generalise about the lived experience of individuals or groups in specific situations, or who encounter similar experiences in life. Such has been the depth of philosophical differences between these two approaches that a degree of incompatibility between the two was long accepted as the status quo. This has been unfortunate for the progression of knowledge in general, but in rehabilitation, and rehabilitation nursing in particular, it has been extremely counterproductive.

The situation is changing, however, and changing fast, with both paradigms now appreciating that the other has valuable but different insights to offer the discipline. This rapproachement is most vividly displayed in two important publications for the discipline of rehabilitation. These are Goodwill, Chamberlain and Evans' (1997) second edition of the textbook, *Rehabilitation of the Physically Disabled Adult*, and Brown's (1997) second edition of the reader *Quality of Life for Handicapped People*. In the first text (Goodwill, et al. 1997), the chapter by Hunter on the nature and use of outcomes, indices and measurements is a testament to the degree of progress that the quantitative analysis of outcomes measurement has made over the last 10 years. Although the chapter is predominantly concerned with the measurement of client progression over the period of rehabilitation input, concern is continually raised about the abstracted nature of some measures and the need for the client's perspective to be fully appreciated. This opinion is also addressed in the discussion by Cummins in the second text (Brown, 1997) in relation to the measurement of quality of life. The ability of rehabilitation to affect the quality of life of both the client and their carer is at the core of the practice of rehabilitation care. The ability to measure that effect has traditionally been a difficult task that has been centred upon the identification of specific aspects of the concept, such as those isolated by Blunden (1987) as concerning 'physical wellbeing', 'cognitive wellbeing', 'material wellbeing' and 'social wellbeing' and by Felce and Perry (1997) as concerning 'physical wellbeing', 'emotional wellbeing', 'material wellbeing', 'productive wellbeing' and 'social wellbeing'. The operationalisation of such aspects as these led to a situation where quality of life could be gauged in numerical terms, which had little or no meaning to the lived experiences of those individuals that were measured. Hence Cummins (1997) argues that the opinions of the clients and their carers should be directly addressed by means of qualitative research.

The situation is, therefore, that in both these prestigious texts, arguments are being put forward calling for a far more eclectic approach to the methods used in rehabilitation research. The obvious question therefore, is how does this effect the practice of rehabilitation nursing research? The answer is, of course, that nurses need to be well versed in both approaches. Nurses have traditionally been strong in the qualitative paradigm, where their closeness to the client and carers has made them more open to the sorts of issues that are best addressed by these methods. Nurses must begin to appreciate the value of quantitative methods to the same degree, to appreciate that such methods are of value in determining policy issues regarding care regimes, and to understand the importance of the ability to generalise on results gained by formal sampling techniques. What is being argued for is that nurses widen their control of research enterprise to the widest sphere of methods, so that no questions that relate to rehabilitation nursing are seen to be outside their methodological remit.

Given that only a minority of clinically-based nurses can be directly involved in research projects on the scale envisaged by research studies funded on a full-time basis, the responsibilities of clinical nurses lie in directly associated areas. The first is research awareness, the second, research participation and the third, an understanding of the limits of research for clinical practice.

The concept of research awareness is now a familiar one. The belief that both a knowledge of research findings and an understanding of such findings is the underpinning of the knowledgeable practitioner is embedded in the present pre-registration nursing curriculum. The concept of the knowledgeable doer subsumes the two aspects defined above, in that the nurse should both be aware of and have an understanding of research results. This chapter and text as a whole supports this belief and assumes that such knowledge that is required to understand research findings is to be found in its readers.

There is, however, a problem in the awareness aspect of the concept. With the completion of a newly registered nurse's pre-registration education, it is not uncommon to observe a tailing off amongst such nurses in their dedication to reading journals when new information is required. This is understandable given that the new and enormous pressures of a first year staff nurse post do not allow for the time that was available during training. However, habits once lost are hard to regain. It is therefore the responsibility of the senior nurse and the mentor of the newly qualified nurse, to constantly foster such research mindedness in the care delivery, by themselves being aware of the latest research in their field of nursing. This is not difficult to sustain – a simple journal club where each member scans a particular journal to search for relevant articles is not overly time-consuming and the published results can be most beneficial. Hence, in rehabilitation where the number of journals is relatively few, this is an avenue well worth travelling.

Research participation implies that nurses should be involved in research. Being involved in research does not mean that every D Grade should commence a PhD! Being involved in research means two things. First, where projects are in progress, being an active and enthusiastic participant, and secondly, being involved in the analysis of care delivery to such an extent that the need for research in a particular problem can be perceived by the nurse.

The first of these levels of involvement can be perceived at various levels. The first and most obvious is the participation in formal research programmes that may exist, but the idea goes further. For example, many studies are retrospective, that is, researchers look back on care that has been given and associated outcomes of clients that have been displayed. Hence, the accurate and correct (and often laborious) completion of documentation is essential if such research is to be valid. Similarly, the accurate scoring of clients on the various scales that many units use to estimate function and other impairments can be central, not only to the validity of such studies, but may also go some way to justifying not only the nurses' input, but in some cases, the validity of a rehabilitation unit's existence.

Lastly, the nurse should be aware of the limits of research. This is not just associated with an awareness of methodology but also with the ethical limits of research studies. The most important limitation is the degree to which research findings should influence practice. There is no doubt that practice should be research-based but the degree to which individual client care should be research-led, is an aspect in which it is more difficult to be categorical. The difficulty arises from the importance of randomised controlled trials (RCTs) and the particular care of individual clients. For example, the RCTs of stroke units versus other areas demonstrate that clients will have on average a better outcome on stroke units than in other areas. This is not the same as saying a particular client will do better on a stroke unit than in another area. The results of an RCT indicate which course of action is generally best, this does not mean that such a course is best in all cases. There may be very good reasons why such a course of action may not be the best and hence should not be taken. The essential point here is that nurses should not lose sight of their clinical judgement. Research evidence should be used in association with clinical expertise and never as a substitute for it.

The second limitation with research evidence is that it must be accepted that what may successfully benefit one client will not necessarily do so for all. Research evidence provides the nurse with a set of options as to the correct course of treatment. The actual decision to implement a course of action will once again depend upon the clinical judgement of the nurse. For example, there are now various forms of interventions for the successful treatment of pressure ulcers. The decision between any two or three of these will depend upon the particular circumstances of the client. The nurse must use their clinical expertise to exercise judgement over which is the correct course of action.

The third area of limitation is the ethics of client participation in research. As has been argued elsewhere in this book, nurses' 24-hour responsibility gives then an insightful knowledge of client and carer which is greater than that of any of the other team members. Such knowledge must be put to use in decisions about whether a client should participate in research activities if their own decision-making powers are compromised. Similarly, it is part of the nurse's responsibility to ensure that should the client and carer be able to make such decisions themselves, then the nurse should equip them with the knowledge and skill to make and communicate their decision.

As can be seen, these two features are examples of the nurse's advocate and empowerment roles respectively. Such roles are well understood by nurses. The application of them in the sphere of research is centred upon the concept of consent. The ability of a client and their carer to participate in a trial is their decision. The nurse must offer advice, if asked to inform their decision and the decision must be respected not only by the nurses but by the other team members. This chapter has not set out to attempt to cover the content of the many research method textbooks that exist, some examples of which are offered at the end of the chapter. What has been considered are the issues that have implications for nurses in rehabilitation. What is hoped is that the issues raised will open debate and discussion amongst both students and staff concerning the way forward, and the appropriate paths that nurses should take, being aware of the limitations that exist.

References

Brown, R. ed (1997) *Quality of Life for Handicapped People*, 2nd edn. Cheltenham: Stanley Thornes (Publishers) Ltd.

Blunden, R. (1987) Quality of life in persons with disabilities: issues in the development of services. In *Quality of Life for Handicapped People*, 2nd edn, ed. Brown, R. Cheltenham: Stanley Thornes (Publishers) Ltd.

Cummins, R. (1997) In *Quality of Life for Handicapped People*, 2nd edn, ed. Brown, R. Cheltenham: Stanley Thornes (Publishers) Ltd.

Felce, D. & Perry, J. (1997) In *Quality of Life for Handicapped People*, 2nd edn, ed. Brown, R. Cheltenham: Stanley Thornes (Publishers) Ltd.

Feigenson, J. (1981) Stroke rehabilitation. *Stroke*, **12**, 373–375.

Gibbon, B. (1992) The role of the nurse in rehabilitation. *Nursing Standard*, **6**, 32–35.

Goodwill, C., Chamberlain, A. & Evans, C. (1997) *Rehabilitation of the Physically Disabled Adult*, 2nd edn. Cheltenham: Stanley Thornes (Publishers) Ltd.

Gordon, D., Swain, K., Basta, S. (1996) Developing research priorities for rehabilitation nursing. *Rehabilitation Nursing Research*, **5**, 60–66.

Nolan, M., Nolan, J. & Mason, H. (1997) *Preparation for Multi-professional/multi-agency Health Care Practice*. English National Board Research Highlights Number 28. London: English National Board.

O'Connor, S. (1993) Nursing and rehabilitation: the interventions of nurses in stroke patient care. *Journal of Clinical Nursing*, **2**, 29–34.

Orem, R. (1991) *Nursing: Concepts and Practice*, 4th edn. New York: MacGraw-Hill

Waters, K. & Luker, K. (1996) Staff perspectives on the role of the nurse in rehabilitation wards for elderly people. *Journal of Clinical Nursing*, **5**, 105–114.

Worlow, C. et al (1996) *Stroke: A Practical Guide to Management*. London: Blackwell Science.

Further reading

Burges, R. (1984) *In the Field: an Introduction to Field Research*. London: Allen & Unwin.

Bryman, A. (1988) *Quality and Quantity in Social Research*. London: Unwin-Hyman.

Bryman, A. & Burgess, R. (1994) *Analysing Qualitative Data*. London: Routledge.

Cresswell, J. (1996) *Research Design*. Newbury: Sage Publications.

Denzin, N. & Lincoln, Y. (1994) *Handbook of Qualitative Research*. Thousand Oaks: Sage Publications.

Mays, N. & Pope, C. (1995) Rigour and qualitative research. *British Medical Journal*, **311**, 109–112.

Polit, D. & Hungler, B. (1995) *Nursing Research: Principles and Practices*, 5th edn. Philadelphia: J.B. Lippencott Co.

Pope, C. & Mays, N. (1995) Reaching the parts other methods cannot reach: an introduction to qualitative methods in health and health services research. *British Medical Journal*, **311**, 42–45.

Riley, J. (1996) *Getting the Most From Your Data*, 2nd edn. England: The Cromwell Press.

Sapsford, R. & Abbott, P. (1992) *Research Methods for the Caring Professions*. Buckingham: Oxford University Press.

Strauss, A. & Corbin, J. (1990) *Basics of Qualitative Research: Grounded Theory Procedures and Techniques*. Thousand Oaks: Sage Publications.

Talbot, L. (1995) *Principles and Practice of Nursing Research*. St Louis: Mosby Yearbook, Inc.

Useful addresses and resources

ACE/ACCESS Centre
1 Broadbent Road
Watersheddings
Oldham
OL1 4HU
(Email: Ace-access@dial.pipex.com)

Disablement Employment Advisors
Local: Usually via Job Centre.

Headway
National Head Injuries Association
Nottingham
NG1 1EW
(*Leaflets, books, information*)

History of Medicine Museum
Science Museum
London SW7 2DD

North American Nursing Diagnosis Association
1211 Locust Street
Philadelphia
PA 19107
USA

Queen Mary's Hospital Museum
(Artificial Limbs)
Roehampton
London SW15

RCN Rehabilitation Nurses' Forum
20 Cavendish Square
London
W1M 0AB

Stroke Association
CHSA House
Whitecross Street
London EC1Y 8JJ
(*Leaflets, information*)

Wellcome Institute for the History of Medicine
183 Euston Road
London NW1

A video is available entitled 'Hidden Disabilities' from Northwick Park and St Marks NHS Trust. This is a 15-minute presentation giving practical advice to clinicians who communicate with patients with disabilities.

Resources
The internet is rapidly developing and is a useful source of information about assessment in rehabilitation and nursing. Practitioners with access to the internet can try using the search engines available to find a wealth of information.

The following web pages are very useful for details of rehabilitation assessment.

http://www.rehabnurse.org
The Association of Rehabilitation Nurses website. There is a lot of very useful information on this site and links to other sites of related interest.

http://www.healthatoz.com
A useful search engine for health related subjects.

http://www.altavista.digital.com

A general search engine but it often produces more references and links than specific health search engines. Try entering search words such as [rehabilitation + assessment] or [assessment + stroke]. Other searches such as [dysphagia] will produce a wealth of documents and further links.

http:www.ahcpr.gov/

This is the website of the Agency for Health Care Policy and Research in the United States. There are a number of publications including clinical guidelines that are available and of interest to rehabilitation nurses such as incontinence, low back problems, cardiac rehabilitation, stroke and pressure ulcers.

http://www.medlib.com/ahcpr/ psrehab/ahcprtoc.htm.

This has the text of the post stroke rehabilitation clinical guidelines.

http://cais.com/navic/

This is the website of 'National Rehabilitation Information Centre (NARIC) – a national database of rehabilitation-related information in the USA. Made up of research papers, booklists and journal articles, the site averages over 200 new documents per month.

http://codi.buffalo.edu/

This is a collection of resources from community to international level: there are a wide range of documents and statistics available.

http://www.who.int/mnh/icidh/icidh. htm

This is the website with the latest information on WHO's International Classification of Impairments, Activities and Participation Commission (ICIDH-2).

http://www.dysphagia.com

This is a collection of resources regarding swallowing and swallowing disorders

List of NANDA approved nursing diagnoses (1994)

(Reproduced with kind permission from North American Nursing Diagnosis Association)

Activity intolerance
Activity intolerance, risk for
Adaptive capacity, decreased: intracranial
Adjustment, impaired
Airway clearance, ineffective
Aspiration, risk for
Body image disturbance
Body temperature, altered, risk for
Bowel incontinence
Breastfeeding, ineffective
Breastfeeding, interrupted
Breastfeeding, effective
Cardiac output, decreased
Caregiver role strain
Caregiver role strain, risk for
Communication, impaired verbal
Community coping, potential for enhanced
Community coping, ineffective
Confusion, acute
Confusion, chronic
Constipation
Constipation, colonic
Constipation, perceived
Coping, defensive
Coping, family: potential for growth
Coping, ineffective family: compromised
Coping, ineffective family: disabling
Coping, ineffective individual
Decisional conflict (specify)
Denial, ineffective
Diarrhea
Disuse syndrome, risk for
Diversional activity deficit
Dysreflexia
Energy field disturbance

Environmental interpretation syndrome, impaired
Family processes, altered: alcoholism
Family processes, altered
Fatigue
Fear
Fluid volume deficit
Fluid volume deficit, risk for
Fluid volume excess
Gas exchange, impaired
Grieving, anticipatory
Grieving, dysfunctional
Growth and development, altered
Health maintenance, altered
Health-seeking behaviors (specify)
Home maintenance management, impaired
Hopelessness
Hyperthermia
Hypothermia
Incontinence, functional
Incontinence, reflex
Incontinence, stress
Incontinence, total
Incontinence, urge
Infant behavior, disorganized
Infant behavior, disorganized, risk for
Infant behavior, organized: potential for enhanced
Infant feeding pattern, ineffective
Infection, risk for
Injury, perioperative positioning: risk for
Injury, risk for
Knowledge deficit (specify)
Loneliness, risk for

Management for therapeutic regimen, community: ineffective

Management of therapeutic regimen, families: ineffective

Management of therapeutic regimen, individual: effective

Management of therapeutic regimen, individuals: ineffective

Memory, impaired

Mobility, impaired physical

Noncompliance (specify)

Nutrition, altered: less than body requirements

Nutrition, altered: more than body requirements

Nutrition, altered: risk for more than body requirements

Oral mucous membrane, altered

Pain

Pain, chronic

Parent/infant/child attachment, altered: risk for

Parental role conflict

Parenting, altered

Patenting, altered, risk for

Peripheral neurovascular dysfunction, risk for

Personal identity disturbance

Poisoning, risk for

Post-trauma response

Powerlessness

Protection, altered

Rape-trauma syndrome

Rape-trauma: compound reaction

Rape-trauma syndrome: silent reaction

Relocation stress syndrome

Role performance, altered

Self-care deficit, bathing/hygiene

Self-care deficit, dressing/grooming

Self-care deficit, feeding

Self-care deficit, toileting

Self-esteem, disturbance

Self-esteem, chronic low

Self-esteem, situational low

Self-mutilation, risk for

Sensory/perceptual alteration (specify)

Sexual dysfunction

Sexuality patterns, altered

Skin integrity, impaired

Skin integrity, impaired, risk for

Sleep pattern disturbance

Social interaction, impaired

Social isolation

Spiritual distress (distress of the human spirit)

Suffocation, risk for

Swallowing, impaired

Thermoregulation, ineffective

Though processes, altered

Tissue integrity, impaired

Tissue perfusion, altered (specify type) renal, cerebral, cardiopulmonary, gastrointestinal, peripheral

Trauma, risk for

Unilateral neglect

Urinary elimination, altered

Urinary retention

Ventilation, inability to sustain spontaneous ventilatory weaning response, dysfunction

Violence, risk for: self-directed or directed at others

The Rehabilitation Nurses' Forum

In 1988, at a study day, June Bendall (Senior Nurse at the Wolfsen Rehabilitation Centre in Wimbledon) and myself discovered that we were not the only rehabilitation nurses in the UK experiencing difficulties with our role. We identified the need for a forum in which nurses interested in rehabilitation could share ideas and support each other. Following a number of informal meetings, we set up a special interest group with the Royal College of Nursing and then in 1993, became the Rehabilitation Nurses' Forum. Acceptance by the RCN has, I feel, given the group a higher status.

Philosophy of the Forum
Rehabilitation Nurses believe that:

- they should be building on their knowledge base and participating in research relevant to rehabilitation
- rehabilitation should commence at the onset of illness
- an interdisciplinary approach is essential if rehabilitation based on goal-planning is to achieve the best outcome for the client and family
- effectiveness and continuity in rehabilitation can only be achieved through the provision of a 24-hour/7 days a week interdisciplinary service
- clients are people with individual personalities and needs
- they have a role to play in educating nurses and other professions in rehabilitation
- communication is vital to the rehabilitation process

- clients have a right to privacy, dignity and a right to say 'no'
- recreation, leisure and social interaction are important aspects of rehabilitation
- clients are entitled to have a high standard of care from a named registered nurse and named therapists
- a framework is needed to assess, plan and evaluate care which should be developed in partnership with the client and family
- a health promotion focus is necessary to enable them to concentrate on health and wellness rather than disability and illness
- education should be ongoing and must cater for the specialist needs of rehabilitation for staff, clients and relatives.

Aims of the Forum
1. To promote rehabilitation as a key role for all registered nurses
2. To heighten the awareness of other professionals and nurses of the nurse's role in rehabilitation
3. To promote the development of the nurse's role in rehabilitation through research and education
4. To share information, experience and innovations in the field of rehabilitation
5. To provide support for rehabilitation nurses.

Work undertaken by the Forum
- Nursing standards

RCN (1994) *Standards of Care for Rehabilitation Nursing*. Harrow: Scutari The development of standards of care to provide a framework for rehabilitation nurses to develop their own standards in relation to their specific area. The standards cover the areas of professional development, health promotion, interdisciplinary approach, support and counselling, privacy and dignity, the right to say 'no', pain, recreation and leisure, equipment.

Published in 1994 these standards are in the process of being reviewed and being incorporated into a new document detailing the role of the nurse in rehabilitation.

- *The development of regional groups*
  To expand the network, the setting up of regional groups has been instigated by the Forum's committee.

- *Annual conferences*
  The forum has held an annual conference since 1993 which, since 1997, has extended into a two day conference.

- *Membership*
  Membership of the group has risen dramatically in recent years to over 4000 members.

- *Newsletter*
  A regular newsletter is produced to highlight areas of interest regarding rehabilitation.

- *Open learning material*
  An educational package was produced which now needs to be reviewed in light of other developments.

Other work has included the development of a consensus statement with the critical care forum; seconding a resolution at the RCN Congress regarding the client's sexual needs and linking in with other membership groups.

Future work
- The development of a detailed working document on the role of the nurse in rehabilitation
- A directory of educational courses related to rehabilitation nursing
- Re-evaluate the educational package
- Establish international links with other rehabilitation nurses
- Continue to hold an annual conference.

To join the forum you need to be a member of the RCN. There is no charge. Contact the RCN for an application form. As a member you will receive the newsletter and any flyers for conferences, etc.

Sally Davis
Chair, Rehabilitation Nurses' Forum.
Senior Lecturer: Rehabilitation, Rivermead Rehabilitation Centre, Oxford Brookes University, Oxford.

Index